Addiction Recovery Change

A How-To Manual for Successfully Navigating Sobriety

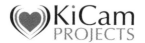

ADAMS RECOVERY CENTER

KiCam
PROJECTS

Cover and book design by Mark Sullivan

ISBN 978-0-9970815-6-5 (paperback)
ISBN 978-0-9970815-7-2 (e-book)

Printed in the United States of America

Published by KiCam Projects
www.KiCamProjects.com

CONTENTS

Seeking Sobriety

When we conceived this book, we wrote it for the person who is contemplating or has just entered substance abuse treatment, sometimes called rehabilitation or "rehab." Almost everyone who abuses substances has hesitation, if not outright fear, about entering treatment. In addition to the stigma attached by many to it, being in treatment can feel like an admission of defeat against something so small—a powder, a drop of liquid, a vapor. These small things can take control of lives, leading people into treatment, where they have to spend time away from their jobs, their friends, their families, and their familiar lives to get things straight. Treatment is scary. Drug use is scary.

Sobriety can be downright terrifying, especially for those who have just completed the beginning portion of their journey out of insobriety.

Therefore, we changed the focus of this book. We wanted to help the person who has just shaken off the cobwebs, probably after spending some time in a detoxification program or in treatment, and finds herself or himself asking, "Now what do I do?"

If that sounds like you, or like someone you care about, we believe this book can help you.

Contrary to what some might say, sobriety isn't a trade secret. You won't join any secret society and learn magic phrases or code words that enable you to remain sober. Quite frankly, sobriety is much simpler than you might realize. Even if you are still in what we call the "pre-contemplation phase," you will gain valuable insight and learn how to use tools for sobriety in this book.

Of course, reading alone won't do it for you. You have to put into practice what you read. Sobriety sounds great on paper, and when applied, it's magnificent. You start to deal with life on your own terms instead of letting life tell you how you're going to be dealt with.

Ask yourself this question: Are you sick and tired of being sick and tired? You've probably been asked that, or you've asked yourself that, in the past—more than once. We bet that the answer is "yes," you *are* sick and tired of being sick and tired. But the effort to get clean and stay clean is overwhelming. In this book, we're going to discuss various stages and phases you will go through and also address common thinking errors. We'll discuss pitfalls, traps, and dangers that unfortunately lurk around many corners. Some of those pitfalls, traps, and dangers come in the form of familiar people, places, and things, so we'll give you tips and strategies for dealing with them. After all, if you're sick and tired of being sick and tired, you are looking for something to help you get on the path of Right Living (a phrase you will hear often and which will be explained later in this book).

One thing needs to be made clear up front, whether you are the person who is entering sustained sobriety, or you are the loved one of someone getting sober, or if you're just a concerned individual who wants to learn more. A sad truth is that most people who get clean use substances again. This is not at all to be considered a failure. Substance abuse is alluring. It is literally stimulating on so many levels. People use again for more reasons than we can list in this book. But using substances again after getting clean does not in any way, shape, or form indicate the person who uses is a failure. It simply means the strategies and tips learned were not sufficient to overcome the desire to use substances. Using again after getting clean gives you a chance to figure out what went wrong and, we hope, to correct that.

There's no sugarcoating the fact that some people who use again could end up dying. No one is immune from the potential for an overdose. If you are under the delusional belief that you cannot end up harmed or dead from using substances, I strongly urge you to spend just a few minutes on the Internet reading the tens of thousands of "It could never happen to me!" stories to find out how many people are no longer with us. Substance abuse destroys.

We'd like to help you avoid becoming an unnecessary casualty.

WHO WE ARE

We are Adams Recovery Center, a separate-gender drug and alcohol treatment program located in Clermont County, Ohio. We offer residential, intensive outpatient, and individual counseling services. Our program is a modified Therapeutic Community running the Hazelden clinical curriculum, and we use the latest evidence-based practices and incorporate cognitive behavioral therapy, rational-emotive behavior therapy, and behavior therapy to maximize client gains in the program. Our inpatient program is designed for an approximate 180-day stay. Our staff includes drug and alcohol counselors and mental health counselors.

When a client has made sufficient evident clinical and personal progress, the client graduates and is referred for aftercare.

Not every client who attends ARC graduates. No program on the planet can guarantee 100 percent success. Many programs exist, and many models exist, but in the end, it's up to the person going through the program to put the work into the program and benefit from what she or he learns.

WHAT QUALIFIES US TO HELP YOU

The staff at Adams Recovery Center comprises individuals who are certified or licensed in various disciplines. All clinical staff hold, at the bare minimum, certification as a chemical dependency counselor in the state of Ohio (Chemical Dependency Counselor Assistant). Most staff are licensed as chemical dependency counselors (Licensed Chemical Dependency Counselor, Level 2 and Level 3), and others hold the Licensed Independent Chemical Dependency Counselor (LICDC). Two staff members hold the LICDC-CS, which is the Clinical Supervisory endorsement—the highest form of chemical dependency licensure in the state of Ohio.

Additionally, several staff are licensed as mental health counselors (LPC) in the state of Ohio. Several of these mental health counselors are under direct supervision as Clinical Residents and are working toward their independent licensure as Licensed Professional Clinical Counselors (LPCC) in the state of Ohio. Our medical coordinator is a Registered Nurse (RN) in the state of Ohio, along with holding a CDCA.

We come from various counseling backgrounds, from a variety of schools of thought. We draw from cognitive behavioral therapy; behavior therapy; rational-emotive behavior therapy; reality therapy; choice therapy; existential/gestalt therapy, etc. We bring a diverse therapeutic orientation to the table, which allows multiple techniques and interventions to be used.

If you tally the years of experience of every clinical professional at Adams Recovery Center, you approach triple digits quickly! We never take a generic, cookie-cutter approach, and we believe this diversity allows us to help clients reach their goals without being placed in a one-size-fits-all box.

As ARC's clinical director, I wrote this book by pulling from the expertise of the entire ARC team. My name is Matthew Rupert, and I've spent more than twenty years working in behavioral health. For the past ten years, my focus has been on addictions. Initially, I wanted to be a therapist helping people with depression, anxiety, and similar issues. I discovered my love for this field because of the people who need the help. They're no different than anyone else. Sure, they have a substance abuse issue, but they're certainly not immoral demons. *They're people.* Some of them have done some really bad things (I've worked with sex offenders, murderers, arsonists, etc.), but they are still *people.* By refusing to judge the person and instead focusing on his or her behaviors, I discovered how intricately woven the behavioral issues are in substance abusers. I also enjoy the personalities in this field. I meet some absolutely fascinating people!

To serve my clients in the best way possible, I earned a Master of Arts in Community Counseling (mental health therapy) from Xavier University in Cincinnati, Ohio. I am a fully licensed Professional Clinical Counselor with supervisory endorsement (LPCC-S) and a Licensed Independent Chemical Dependency Counselor with clinical supervisory endorsement (LICDC-CS), both in the state of Ohio. I have the privilege and honor of being able to work on the behavioral challenges of individuals who present with substance abuse issues or what would be perceived as more "traditional" mental health issues—and in most cases, both.

Despite my credentials and schooling, I don't claim to have all the answers. I don't claim to be able to save everyone's life. I can't take credit for the hard work the client does. I won't pretend I'm the one responsible for change.

I do this work because I love to see someone save her or his own life. Every life is a life worth saving.

Therefore, I'd like you to write down in the next few lines your three biggest challenges in sustained sobriety, whether it's your own sobriety or that of a loved one. In other words, what are the three things you think might lead you or your loved one to use substances again?

1) _____
   _____
   _____

2) _____
   _____
   _____

3) _____
   _____
   _____

Keep those challenges in mind as you read the book. Refer to them in every chapter, and ask yourself, "Are these challenges being addressed?" These are going to be the "Big

Three," and if you work honestly with yourself, they won't be so big once you're done with this book. (These challenges *will* remain insurmountable if you do not honestly work on and address them!)

Throughout these pages, we'll share stories about some of the clients we've seen. To protect those clients, names and some details have been changed. Not every tale you read has a happy ending. These stories are included to illustrate how different every situation is, and that even if you think you understand what someone is going through because you used the same drug(s) or grew up in the same town, you really don't know anything about another person. Every person's experience is different, bar none. You don't know what Billy or Jamie went through unless you happen to *be* Billy or Jamie.

You are the best expert on your own life. We're hoping you'll add your own story at the end of this book, and that it will be one of sustained sobriety.

Reflection Questions

Before we move on, we ask you to reflect on the following:

- What scares you the most about trying to stay sober, or about helping a loved one stay sober?

_____

_____

_____

- What are you most excited about in your new life of sobriety?

  _____

  _____

  _____

- Who are the supporters in your life to whom you can turn for help?

  _____

  _____

  _____

- What is the biggest challenge you have overcome so far on your personal journey?

  _____

  _____

  _____

CHAPTER ONE

Setting Expectations after Treatment

Quite often when we are asked, "What do people do in treatment?" we respond, "They learn how to become and stay sober." This response has, surprisingly to us, been met with skepticism and incredulity. It has been our experience that most of the people who are labeled as supports for the client believe treatment to be a magical place where grand changes will occur with the client. Parents, grandparents, husbands, wives, girlfriends, boyfriends, pastors—you name it— believe that somehow, through the client simply being in the rehabilitation program, a cosmic change will occur for the client and all will be well.

Sadly, we have to disappoint these supporters.

The reality differs from the mental image. In truth, change does occur, but that change occurs over time. We explain that we're working to de-program years, if not decades, of conditioning. The client comes to us with numerous beliefs, some of them highly manipulative and criminal in nature, that led the client to engage in a series of destructive behaviors. It took time to build these harmful, well-defended behaviors, and so it takes time to deconstruct them.

During a client's stay in treatment, we work constantly to destroy the client's defense mechanisms. We want clients to begin to open to the possibility of being something they don't like being: vulnerable. We emphasize that this type of vulnerability will not harm the client; in fact, it is *a healthy risk*. Being vulnerable to hearing someone say, "I care about you," or, "I love you," is healthy and can yield significant personal growth. Shoving a needle full of junk into your vein or slamming an entire bottle of booze, in an effort to cover some pain or trauma, represents the unhealthy risk. We teach that through exposure to healthy risks, life becomes less scary and overwhelming, and in time, our desire and ability to take healthy risks provide much greater rewards than escaping into a drug or a drink.

Embarking on a life of sustained sobriety is a healthy risk. Your friends and family are hoping for positive change in you, and you might worry that you'll let them down. Maybe you already think you're a failure because of your addiction. Maybe you hated yourself when you entered treatment. Maybe you still do to a certain extent.

All of these are normal feelings most people have when they start to come out of active addiction. Therefore, you are not alone. You have millions of brothers and sisters who have gone through, and who are going through, the same things you're experiencing. Like so many brothers and sisters who have struggled as you are struggling, *you can and will succeed at sustained sobriety if you trust the process!*

When we ask someone to trust the process, we are asking him or her to abandon the image he or she holds onto of him- or herself and begin shedding that image, as a snake sheds its skin. We are asking the person to expose his or her true self, or, if the true self is unknown, to allow the true self to be revealed so the true self can be discovered. Addiction takes away so much from us, including our identity, that we no longer recognize who and what we are. In some cases, we don't know if we ever knew who and what we are. Therefore, by trusting the process, we come out of denial and into acceptance.

What Is the Process?

The process is called many things by many people. We do not define it for you. We don't believe the process can be defined by anyone except you. Some say it's God. Others say it's nature. Even more people say it's the entire universe. We've heard people call the process the truth. The process is not something anyone controls. If we learn to accept the fact that the process *simply is,* and that we are a part of it and not masters of it, we stop fighting to control it, and we accept that life will occur. We cannot force our will on the process and demand, insist, or threaten that the process conform to our desires. We already tried that, and sustained addiction was the price we paid.

In short, the process is simply getting from point A to point B. It is comparable to jumping into a river with a strong current. The river isn't deadly in and of itself, but if you fight the current or attempt to alter the path of the river, things might not go the way you envisioned. It might sound mystical, spiritual, or religious. But we remind everyone that there's nothing about the process that is otherworldly. You can think of the process as spiritual or supernatural if that helps. The process represents how things move in this great and wonderful universe in which we are privileged to live. Fighting and bucking against that process results in painful experiences and almost always ends in disaster—hence the analogy of the river. If you fail to trust that the river will take you to your destination, you'll end up spending a lot of energy attempting to change the current to favor you. You might see some short-term gains by doing so, but ultimately, it's a losing battle.

So, What's Next?

It is difficult to prepare for life after treatment, despite everything you might have done to this point. The transition from completely abstinent life in a controlled environment to a life in an environment potentially filled with drugs and alcohol can be difficult. You almost certainly knew and expected that life hadn't changed on the outside while you were in treatment. The same people, places, and things are waiting for you, and unless they, too, have been doing work to help with sustained sobriety, they're not eager to see you change. In some cases, they might belittle, mock, or outright attack you verbally (and sometimes physically) because you have changed your viewpoint regarding your old life. In a nutshell, the life you had before treatment will be drastically changed from the life you have now.

Before you step foot back in your old neighborhood, you should take a moment to inventory your life. Quite often, those in treatment aren't aware of the many toxic and poisonous people, places, and things they had in their lives. As part of your discharge planning from treatment, going through your life and making a careful list of the things that are helpful and harmful is crucial to ensure you don't blindly or even willingly re-enter the areas that you have identified as so-called "triggers."

The word *trigger* is used to explain something that will lead someone in recovery to abusing substances again. This word is used—overused, to be sure—and quite frankly, if you ask anyone who uses substances what his or her triggers are, you will walk away with a huge list. The word *trigger* has become so deeply pounded into our brains as a danger sign that we forget triggers are nothing more than *learned associations*. Therefore, if a trigger can be *learned*, it can be *unlearned*. Ask a nurse what she thinks of when she sees a needle, and then ask someone who is addicted to injecting heroin. Ask a crack cocaine smoker what she thinks of when she sees steel wool, and then ask someone who is a dishwasher. The triggers are learned behavioral pairings, and in and of themselves they have absolutely *zero* control over you and your life.

Because that's the case, why should you worry about triggers?

Triggers are not automatic. Just because you encounter one doesn't mean you will automatically start using, although some people will argue that exposure to *any* trigger immediately will cause you to consume your drug(s) of choice. This mentality has been disproven hundreds of times via experimentation and research. Triggers simply do not exist as they have been portrayed. You will not, for example, immediately and without any control, start using your former drug(s) of choice because of mere exposure to a trigger. You also will not start to break out in a cold sweat, get the shakes, feel violently ill, or otherwise have any negative reaction in the presence of a so-called trigger *unless you already want to use.* The mere presence of the trigger has nothing to do with your substance use; the symptoms you experience in the presence of the trigger are independent of the trigger. It's a behavioral pairing. So, for example, a heroin addict has come to associate needles with using. So when he has a doctor appointment and sees a needle, he might feel the desire to use—even though no heroin is present.

But we know the needle itself is harmless. It has no power. It alone cannot get us high. Yet it's common to make a grossly false association: "Needles are bad, and needles are my trigger." We come to accept that some things absolutely, without question, will lead us to use again.

But we know *trigger* is a fancy word for another one with which you might be familiar: *Excuse.*

Triggers are excuses. Any time you argue, "I can't be around XYZ, because then I'll use," you are making an excuse. You are looking for that situation to occur so that when you do use, you will have an excuse as to why you used. You will avoid responsibility and you will shift the blame. How very convenient life would be if everyone on the planet could simply say, "It wasn't me, it was my trigger. I have no control over my trigger. Oh, woe is me, the trigger made me do it!" We hear this on television, in courtrooms, and even at the grocery store. Everyone—even people who have never used drugs—seems to have an excuse as to why they do certain things.

We suggest you view triggers as what they really are— excuses—and realize you will never escape the things you've falsely labeled as permission for you to use. These excuses you have gain their power from you. Once you give that excuse your power, you have so much less for yourself.

What about Meetings?

Support meetings are highly beneficial. We absolutely encourage you to find a good support group in which you will be welcomed and can express your thoughts and feelings safely. We strongly encourage you to visit several types of sober support meetings, because everyone has a different set of expectations. Not everyone wants, for example, to attend an Alcoholics Anonymous or Narcotics Anonymous meeting; some people don't care for step-based support groups. *It's OK whether you do or do not.* Some people prefer Secular Sobriety, Rational Recovery, Celebrate Recovery, or simply finding a nonaligned local support group. As long as you are gaining good sober support, you will be in a better place than you used to be.

We do not recommend you replace your life with meeting attendance. By this, we mean some people will say you should attend "90 meetings in 90 days." First, there has been no evidence that attending multiple sober support meetings in a short amount of time demonstrates a decreased desire to abuse substances. As a matter of fact, the evidence shows the more meetings one attends in a short period of time, the higher risk the person has of dropping out of sober support meetings altogether. Also, attending multiple meetings instead of living your life is substituting one addictive pattern for another. Now, instead of doing drugs all the time, you're buried in attending meetings all the time. In order to live a healthy life, you have to *live* your life, not avoid life by hiding out in meetings. Again, we fully encourage you to attend sober support meetings, but we also fully encourage you to live your life and find out what you truly enjoy doing. Don't let one obsession replace another!

A caution: Some sober support meetings are "hunting grounds" for some of their attendees. Some people who attend those meetings prey on new members. These hunters look for those who are vulnerable, and as you can imagine, are eager to form a relationship with someone who shows the slightest bit of kindness. We understand that you might be lonely and you might like the thrill of being given attention from someone. But just because you are out of treatment doesn't mean you are 100 percent good to go. You still need time to work on you. We ask that you seriously ask yourself, "Am I really ready for a relationship?" Even a short-term intimate relationship can be damaging. Be cautious of those who are too eager to be your friend, especially if he or she wants more than that.

Do You Need More Treatment?

Aftercare is something you might have heard mentioned. We strongly encourage clients to engage in an aftercare program, such as intensive outpatient or outpatient programming. This is continued clinical programming that occurs in a nonresidential setting. You don't stay at the facility, but you attend two or three groups per week. This can last anywhere from six to sixteen weeks depending on the program you choose to attend. Clinical programming is not the same thing as a sober support group. Clinical programming is run by clinicians who work with you on areas in which you might need additional help and enable you to build your "staying sober tool chest" so you can better deal with situations that might arise outside of treatment. Aftercare is a great place for anyone transitioning from treatment back to the real world.

• • • BETTY'S STORY • • •

A few years ago, I started my tenure as director of an inpatient rehabilitation facility. On my second day, which was the first day I entered group to observe staff, I witnessed a young lady who was about to present her autobiography.

This has been a staple of our rehabilitation: present one's life story without glorifying or glossing over important portions. It's an opportunity for clients to share and to give others an opportunity to know more about them. Also, it helps promote an atmosphere of honesty and trust.

One young lady, Betty, pulled out her notebook and was going to read her autobiography. Before she began reading, she said, "It's forty-nine pages. I'll go quick." From the back of the room, I asked Betty, "Can I see your notebook for a moment?" I walked up to her, and she handed it to me. I took it from her, walked back to my seat, and said, "Go ahead with your auto." She started to cry. She said, "I can't! I need my notebook!" I responded calmly, "You, and you alone, are the best and only person who knows your entire life history. There's nothing in here you already don't know better than anyone. We trust you. You can do this."

Long story short, she got through it.

And, yes, she was displeased with me.

When she graduated some time later, she came up to me and said, "I never liked what you did to me with my autobiography. But I got through it, and I realized that what you did was to help me. I didn't like you for what you did, but now I understand why, and I wanted to thank you. I also stopped being mad at you."

Betty didn't believe in herself. She didn't believe she had it in her to do what she needed to do. She thought things had to be a certain way, and that was for a lot of things in her life. I asked her, "Did it ever occur to you to do your auto from memory?" She said it hadn't, and because everyone else had read it from a notebook, she assumed, *that was just the way it was.* She also confided in me that up to that point, she was going through the motions but had no intention of changing because everyone else around her had stagnated. She figured, why bother aspiring to new heights?

Betty had fallen victim to a classic thinking error: that is, "Because this is the way I've seen things done, they are done only this way." Betty did not, would not, and *could not* envision doing things differently. And I don't just mean her autobiography.

This reminds me of a story with five monkeys in a cage. The story goes as follows:

A group of scientists placed five monkeys in a cage, and in the middle, a ladder with bananas on top. Every time a monkey went up the ladder, the scientists soaked the rest of the monkeys with cold water. After a while, every time a monkey would start up the ladder, the others would pull it down and beat it up. After some time, no monkey would dare try climbing the ladder, no matter how great the temptation. The scientists then decided to replace one of the monkeys. The first thing this new monkey did was start to climb the ladder. Immediately, the others pulled him down and beat him up. After several beatings, the new monkey learned never to go up the ladder, even though there was no evident reason not to, aside from the beatings. The second monkey was substituted and the same occurred. The first monkey participated in the beating of the second monkey. A third monkey was changed and the same was repeated. The fourth monkey was changed, resulting in the same, before the fifth was finally replaced as well. What was left was a group of five monkeys that continued to beat up any monkey who attempted to climb the ladder. If it was possible to ask the monkeys why they beat up on all those who attempted to climb the ladder, their most likely answer would be, "I don't know. It's just how things are done around here."

Many of us have become like the monkeys. We are doing something because those around us do it, and when we attempt to change what we do, or worse yet, even dare to *think* about doing it a different way, we are scolded, chided, and in some cases, violence is perpetrated upon us. Thus, we end up settling for the status quo and never reaching our potential. We never reach our destination because we have accepted falsehoods about our lives. Betty fell into that trap, but once someone gave her permission to do something different, she had an opportunity to make a critical choice.

Betty chose to be different. Betty chose to do differently. Betty *became* different.

Betty made a choice to empower herself. She remains clean and sober to this day.

Had Betty chosen to remain the same, you can imagine where she'd be right now. She might even be dead. Betty had to make tough choices, look at herself in the mirror, and ask, "Is this all I want out of life?" The answer was a resounding, "No!" Betty's choice to enter a lifestyle of drug use and destruction was ended by Betty's choice to enter a life of sustained sobriety and purpose.

But first, Betty had to enter rehabilitation. She knew she needed help. She couldn't do it on her own. Betty admitted in her autobiography that she felt like a failure. She didn't think she had a problem, and if she did, she could beat it on her own. After all, if she'd gotten into this mess on her own, she could get herself out. She repeatedly fell into the cycle of destruction because she lacked the tools to make an effective change. Betty didn't want to be in treatment because she wanted freedom. Her freedom, however, was what landed her in treatment in the first place.

Betty's struggle continued during her stay in treatment. Faced with the same situations and same people, she rationalized that it would be better to go through motions versus going through changes. Working with her counselor and with the rest of the clients in the program, Betty started to expand her trust. She initially trusted no one, not even herself. When I took away her preprinted autobiography, I wanted to convey the message to her that we trusted her to complete this task. I didn't know Betty at that point, but it was clear that she was nervous and unsure of herself. I took her out of her comfort zone—something she'd done to herself the first time she'd experimented with drugs—and she had to make a choice. She wasn't happy, but she made it through.

When she was graduating, I asked her if it had been a hard choice to enter treatment. She told me it was the hardest decision she'd ever made. I asked her what made it so hard and she told me about her perceived failure in life and how treatment would be a daily reminder of that. I reframed her comment by stating, "Entering treatment would be a daily reminder of your desire to relearn what you unlearned." Betty thought about that, smiled, and agreed. She said that treatment helped her figure out what she needed to figure out, enough to get her up and running.

REFLECTION QUESTIONS

- How do you define "the process" for yourself?

_____

_____

_____

- What have you identified as potential "triggers"?

_____

_____

_____

- If you reframe those triggers as excuses, how does that help you see your life—and your future of sustained sobriety—differently?

_____

_____

_____

CHAPTER TWO

Finding Sober Supports

After exiting treatment, it doesn't matter if you have the best support system in the world or if you don't have anyone to whom you can turn. You will feel all alone regardless of who has or hasn't been supporting you. The sudden change of behavior is bound to alienate those you thought were close to you. Additionally, you find yourself restricted or bored due to the need to stay away from old people, places, and things. When nighttime comes, it seems the darkness closes in and there's nowhere to go, nothing to do, no one to call.

On top of that, you're now dealing with all of the things that came about as a result of your addiction. You may be facing unemployment, homelessness, damaged or destroyed relationships, debt, health problems—the list goes on. The difficulty in your life seems insurmountable. You start to ask questions: What do I do? How do I do it? How long will it take? Will my life ever be normal? Have I screwed myself up completely?

No doubt, this sounds bleak. As desperate as the situation sounds, you know entering the lifestyle of addiction and destruction is what led to these problems in the first place. There will be temptation to abuse substances again.

You'll hear the familiar voices tell you, "It's OK. Go ahead—use. You'll stop caring." You already know the dark road down which drug abuse leads. Never has drug abuse led you to salvation, never has it led you to a permanent state of happiness, and never has drug abuse been a solution on any level. Any perceived benefits from drug abuse are extremely short-term, and there's always a massive cost.

In the previous chapter, we encouraged you to have a strong sober support system. The more sober supports you have—they could be a sponsor, sober friends, parents, a spouse, a priest or pastor, a nurse or doctor—the better the chances for increasing your sustained sobriety. There's a catch, however: You might have come to believe that no one understands you because they haven't been through what you have been through.

A common misconception is that only those who have been through your experience are capable of understanding you or helping you. For some reason, addiction is the only professional field in which it is believed that the counselors are former addicts and that anyone who works in the field has deep, personal issues with drug use. The truth is, a large percentage of individuals who work in substance abuse do not have a former or current addiction. People enter this field because they want to help. It is our experience that those who have a personal experience with substance abuse are no better at helping than those who have been sober their entire lives. Familiarity with an issue does not guarantee an increased demonstrated level of competence. As a matter of fact, some who have a former substance abuse issue might over-empathize or blur boundaries and engage in unethical behavior. This is borne out of a desire to help, undoubtedly, but it ends up costing both the helper and the helped.

Helpers are not supposed to be in the profession of giving advice, because advice is not what you need. Think about the worst times in your life. You probably wanted someone to point the way out of your troubles and into safety. More than likely, that never happened. You would have given anything for someone to come along and show you how to escape. Now, think about those who offered advice and ask yourself if they truly helped or if they were just talking so they could *sound* like they were helping. Helping professionals are in the business to offer feedback and possibly clarification, but not to solve your problems for you. No one can do that.

One of the most important things to remember is that you are *not* alone despite what you might believe. Millions of people have, or have had, issues with substance abuse. Although these numbers are unfortunately high, they demonstrate how much substance abuse permeates society. Substance abuse does not discriminate based on gender, race, religion, social status, education level, etc. You will find many people who are looking to form social relationships to keep themselves grounded in sobriety.

The first step, of course, is opening up the lines of communication with those who are looking for social sober supports, just as you are. Some people have social anxiety and don't do well interacting with strangers. The good news is that with today's technology, those who have social anxiety can reach out to people on computer forums and messaging boards, chats, and texting applications, in addition to simply making good old-fashioned telephone calls (if face-to-face interaction is overwhelming). Also, reaching out to mental health agencies and professionals in your area will, at the very least, put you in touch with those who are able to offer social sober support.

• • • JACK'S STORY • • •

Jack came to treatment after hitting what he called "the bottom of the barrel." Jack is a forty-two-year-old male who had started using methamphetamine ("meth") at the age of twenty-nine. He was using so much that all of his teeth had rotted away. By the time he was thirty-one, he looked like he was in his early fifties. Jack's health had deteriorated rapidly.

Jack was an outstanding client. He truly hated the lifestyle he was living, hated using meth, and had nothing but the desire to get clean, stay clean, and change just about everything in his life. He put in a tremendous effort, challenged his demons, and was on the path to sustained sobriety. If a model client exists, Jack was it. Well-liked by staff and his peers in the program, Jack did what he needed to and then some.

But Jack was terrified. He was scared because he had nowhere to go, no one to support him, and no job. In short, Jack's support system was nonexistent. He wanted desperately to avoid the old people, places, and things, but without so much as a single person who was sober support, Jack's prospects of sustained sobriety were bleak.

With Jack's permission, Jack's counselor and other program staff started to work with community support systems to help Jack find appropriate sober housing. Jack met with three housing agencies and managers to find a sober home where he could transition. Within two weeks, Jack had lined up sober housing. Additionally, Jack met with an employment specialist in the community who helped him start the process of getting his birth certificate so he could get a state ID, which in turn would help Jack secure a job.

Jack hadn't attended any sober support meetings during treatment, but he soon started to attend regularly. Jack stated he wasn't a fan of the messages from the sober support groups, but he attended in order to meet sober community supports. Jack understood the importance of networking and learning about the major resources in the community. Jack became a regular at every type of sober support meeting and quickly filled his notebook with names, numbers, and addresses.

By the time Jack's graduation came, he had secured sober housing, received his state ID, had leads for employment at a local construction company, and had been invited to several sober support functions. Jack joked, "I have a social calendar now!"

Jack's story is noteworthy because it not only illustrates a strong desire to get clean and stay sober, but it also shows the value of putting in the necessary work to ensure a strong sober support network. Jack knew the clinical work he had done was only a portion of what had to happen in order to get and keep him on the right path. Without strong sober supports, Jack's chances of maintaining his sobriety were low. Jack also took ownership of his sobriety. He knew he did not have the right support network. Instead of using that as an excuse, Jack used that as motivation.

REFLECTION QUESTIONS

- Who has been your biggest supporter(s) during your work toward sobriety?

_____

_____

_____

- What has been your biggest motivation to *become* sober?

_____

_____

_____

- What has been your biggest motivation to *stay* sober?

_____

_____

_____

- What are the things you're afraid to lose if you don't stay sober?

_____

_____

_____

CHAPTER THREE

Assessing Your Relationships

This chapter can be summarized in one sentence: You need to seriously evaluate and critically analyze your relationships with people, places, and things to determine what you must avoid.

Some of the people in your life who were present when you were getting high are toxic. They are cancerous individuals who can't wait for you to come back into their "welcoming arms" so they can start to use with you again. They miss you. They don't miss you like a friend misses you. They miss you because you are a using buddy. You got high with them. They want to do that with you again.

Take an inventory of the people you know. How many would not object to using with you again? Now, ask yourself: Are they truly happy? We bet these people are completely miserable, so remember the saying: Misery loves company. Those who are wallowing in the quagmire of substance abuse haven't risen to the level they want. As a result, they swim near the bottom and urge you to join them. Unfortunately, all you can do at the bottom is drown. There's no salvation there, no freedom, just you and a few others swimming in a pit of desolation and despair.

The good news for them is, you're doing it together. But you're going to sink fast.

Continue taking inventory of the people with whom you used to use. Think about what sorts of behaviors in which they'd engage. Think about what they would say, what they would do, all to encourage you to keep using with them. A familiar cry we hear in bars is, "Just have one more drink with me!" It's a desperate attempt to get someone to keep using, because the person who says that is empty inside. He has nothing else to do except sit on a bar stool and keep filling himself with alcohol. He thinks the drug fills the void inside. He begs you to stay and be just as miserable as he is. When he finally crawls home, he goes alone. He is staving off the inevitable, and he hopes you'll be a party to that.

Think about the heroin user who begs, "Just do one more cap with me!" She has absolutely nothing going for her, so she fills her life with drugs. Drug use has become her way of life. Now she's begging you to stay with her and use with her, because in her misery, she has company.

Think about the people with whom you go to parties. They love to get high there! There will be drugs there, and alcohol, too. And with those two things often comes unprotected sex. Your party "friends" seem to believe that if they black out and can't remember what they did, then it didn't happen. No problem, right?

These types of people are *enablers*. They do not care if you have a substance abuse issue. They see you as just another passenger on the ride, and if you fall off the vehicle and get run over, oh well, that's your problem. They'll find someone else to go along with them.

Some people, however, aren't enabling you because they're lonely. Some enable you because when you're using, you're difficult to deal with. Therefore, they will give you money and sometimes drugs just so you'll leave them alone. These people are sick and tired of dealing with you. Therefore, they give you whatever it takes to get you to go away. They don't care about your welfare or well-being; they just want you to leave them alone.

Others enable you by selling you drugs and alcohol. Your dope boy and bartender don't care if you live or die; they'll always have other customers. They'll tell you it's OK to keep using, that you really aren't hurting anyone by your ongoing substance abuse, and in the end, it's your body to do with as you want. These arguments might sound compelling, and you might give in. But your dealers aren't telling you the truth. They just want to sell you a product. They'll lie and twist the truth so you'll buy just one more hit.

Keep in mind that your dealer was *never* your friend. Your dealer was a businessperson selling you something, pure and simple. You are nothing more than another business transaction. Friends don't sell other friends poison and then rationalize that sale by saying, "Hey, you're a grown-up, you made your own choice to buy it. I only provided a service." If that sounds like criminal thinking and rationalizing, you're doing far better than you might give yourself credit for.

• • • SAM'S STORY • • •

Sam's tale is much like Jack's story from the previous chapter. Sam's sober support network didn't exist.

Sam had his own house, but he was in a relationship with a woman who also lived there. Sam also had some friends who lived in the house with him, and although Sam was the official owner of the house, he couldn't kick the others out due to some technicality with the law. On the positive side, Sam had a job that provided financial means. But Sam was worried about living in the house with these people. His girlfriend still used heroin, and his friends used just about anything they could find.

Sam didn't have anywhere else to live. His closest relative was ten hours away, and all his friends had used drugs or alcohol to excess. His options made Sam's sustained sobriety questionable.

Sam's counselor told him, "You have many choices, but you're saying you don't. I wonder if you truly have no choices or if the choices you do have are simply unpleasant to you." Sam admitted he didn't like the choices he had (i.e., live in a homeless shelter, live in a halfway house, get a sober housing apartment, or return to his home). Sam wanted an ideal solution, but one did not exist. Sam wanted his own house back, but he knew that would be a lengthy and costly legal fight.

Eventually, Sam had to make a hard choice, and it was not one he wanted to make. He elected to rent a small apartment. He also threw away his cell phone and bought a new one with a new phone number attached to it, one he gave only to his supervisor at work and to sober support networks. Sam didn't go back to his house, not even to pick up clothing or personal items, in case someone might follow him to his apartment.

Sam had the bills from his house transferred to his apartment. Without electric, heat, water, and Internet service, Sam's girlfriend and friends moved out. Within six months of graduation from treatment, Sam was able to retake his house. Sam reported that his old friends and girlfriend tried to move back in once Sam retook possession of his house, but he stood his ground and they didn't bother him anymore.

Sam had to make difficult choices and he had to give up something that was dear to him: his house. But through persistence and trusting that things would work—trusting the process— Sam regained what he had worked toward in the first place.

The Choice Is Yours

One of the things we hear in addiction treatment is, "I don't have anywhere to go! I have to move back home!" We tell our clients that you always have a choice, but you might not like the choice. We understand it's hard to give up everything you know, but if the cost of familiarity is your ongoing sobriety, then the difficulty is worth it. If you spend time evaluating your options by going back to an old place where drugs and the drug-seeking lifestyle are the norm, you know how that probably will turn out. The same can be said about going back to live with a person who is not sober. You're not getting sober support, because the people who surround you won't let up. They will do anything and everything to drag you down into their misery; if they're not happy, they don't want you to be, either.

Therefore, a hard choice might be made to pack it all up, move into a halfway house or a homeless shelter, or simply shred your cell phone and move across the country. Difficult choices await you in sustained sobriety—that much is certain. But do you remember how difficult it was to live the drug lifestyle? How difficult has that journey been, every step of the way? Ask yourself what benefits you derived from ongoing insobriety and determine how rewarding it was to be high all the time. Take an honest inventory of your life while you were at the bottom of your insobriety and evaluate the pros and cons.

Reflection Questions

- What difficult choices are you facing in your new life?

  _____

  _____

  _____

- What options exist for you? What appeals to you about each one? What does *not* appeal to you?

  _____

  _____

  _____

- What are three things you're looking forward to in your new sober lifestyle?

  _____

  _____

  _____

- Why is it important to you to make a hard choice instead of risking a return to insobriety?

  _____

  _____

  _____

CHAPTER FOUR

Breaking Free of Codependence

One young client wanted desperately to get clean and stay sober, but he was haunted by the facts that everyone in his family used drugs; his neighborhood was well-known for being rife with drug dealers; and everyone he knew either sold drugs, used drugs, or both. He never had a legitimate job, and he had dropped out of school in the ninth grade. He "dabbled" in marijuana, but his main drug was crack cocaine. At the age of twenty-two, he wanted to turn his life around because, as he said, "I've been to the absolute middle of nowhere and I kept on going. There's nothing there." After his time in treatment, he was not looking forward to his graduation.

He had rationalized that, no matter what gains he made in treatment, those gains would be tossed out the window as soon as he went back home. He had no money, so he couldn't get his own place. He didn't know anyone outside of his small, two-block neighborhood. He had no contacts to point him in the right direction. We were able to bring in support groups, sober members of the community, and an employment services programmer. All of them together helped the client build a support network so he could start a new life. In his words: "I'm not starting over; hell, I never even started. This *is* my start." He was able to earn a state ID card, get a copy of his birth certificate, file for a Social Security card, and connect with the owner of a halfway house. Upon graduation, he lived at the house and found a part-time job within two days. One month later, he was working full time and was saving money for his own apartment. Two months later, he was ready to move into his own place. As he said, "I can be my own man for the first time in my life."

Less than one week after he secured his own apartment, he started using crack again.

He explained that he had missed his mom and his brothers, so he started to hang out with them. He said: "They were pissed off that I was sober. They hated the fact that I wasn't the same kid I used to be. They made me feel guilty and made me feel like I wasn't part of the family. They all smoke crack, so, to fit in and be part of my family, I smoked, too." The more we talked with him, the more obvious it was that he needed additional supports in his life. We worked with him on a short-term basis to help him reconnect with sober supports in the community. It took him about a year of on-again/off-again drug usage to finally stop using for good. He enrolled in a community college, earned a two-year degree in computer science, and now has a successful career as a computer technician.

The last time we heard from him, he shared that it was hard not being in touch with his family. But he said he voluntarily severed ties with them because they were not supportive of him being sober. They were actually angry with him because he had, in their words, turned his back on them and now he thought he was better than they were. Although he was saddened by this, he knew he needed to do what he did for himself and he could not be responsible for the feelings and thoughts of his family. He therefore voluntarily cut ties with his family, earned his degree, and moved several hours away to ensure he could keep his life on track.

This story is even richer when you know the background. The young man and his family were involved in criminal enterprise. They all bought, sold, and used crack cocaine. The family also had a history of petty theft and robbery. The family supported itself financially through stealing from stores and people's houses and, of course, selling drugs. Because the entire family was involved in criminal activity, the family had to, as the client stated "watch out for each other, and we had each other's backs. We didn't snitch. That would kill us." The family stole together and worked their criminal activities together. The client said, "Even if you were sick or not in the mood, you had to help. They'd make you feel guilty and scream at you and say stuff like, 'You don't care about us,' or, 'Why don't you love us to help us out?' You helped out, even when you didn't feel like it, or else you got into fights."

The family had a problem that is unfortunately common in most tales of addiction. The family has a strong streak of codependence. Many people use this term incorrectly when they mean "dependence" versus "codependence." In a nutshell, codependence is when two or more people have an excessive and unhealthy emotional and/or mental reliance on another person(s). Usually it's two people who are codependent on each other. Sometimes codependent relationships are called "relationship addiction" because the behaviors displayed in the codependent relationship have the same unhealthy and addictive characteristics as substance abuse. To help you understand what a codependent relationship looks like, below are some characteristics to watch out for. (Note that the following are not exhaustive.)

The thought or belief that you cannot exist without the other person. In a healthy relationship, when two people genuinely love each other, they want to be together, and the thought of losing the other is tremendously saddening. But unlike in a healthy relationship, the codependent person (CDP) actually believes he or she will be unable to function on any level without the other person. The codependent person believes he will be less than a person without the other.

Caregiving vs. partnership. The CDP acts as a caregiver instead of an equal partner. This looks like the role a parent plays for a child.

Lack of emotional responsibility. CDPs will say things such as, "I'm not going to be happy unless you're happy," or, "You being angry makes me angry." Healthy people are able to take responsibility for their own feelings instead of putting ownership on others.

Rescuing. CDPs have a sense of responsibility and duty to "save" their partners. The CDP sees the other person as someone who requires intervention, almost constantly, to ensure the survival and ongoing positive health (mental, emotional, physical) of the other person. This is sometimes expressed as, "I can fix him," or, "I'll save her from herself."

Lack of personal value. CDPs usually feel the need to be in a relationship in order to have a sense of value. CDPs will be in *any* sort of relationship, even an abusive one, because a CDP does not believe he or she can be alone. Being alone equates to being a failure.

Lack of assertiveness. CDPs will "take what they get" and not stick up for themselves. They believe they are not entitled, nor do they deserve, to be treated in a way that would depict a healthy, caring, loving relationship.

People-pleasing. CDPs will go out of their way to ensure everyone else's wants and needs are addressed, but CDPs will not make much, if any, effort to ensure their own needs are met. CDPs believe they don't matter, and in most cases, they believe having any wants and needs is selfish and unnecessarily self-indulgent.

Issues with control. CDPs have issues with control. CDPs will do what they can to bring order and control to the life of another person, and, in return, the person whose life they are helping bring order and control to brings order and control to the life of the CDP. Control, in the perception of the CDP, brings order to the chaos because control is a need for other people to behave in a certain way so that the CDP feels OK.

Obsessive thinking. CDPs will worry to an unhealthy level about the thoughts, feelings, and actions of another person. CDPs will believe that their partner is cheating on them when the partner isn't present or that the partner no longer loves them. CDPs' obsession is rooted in deep denial about the reality of another person's thoughts, feelings, and behaviors.

Low self-esteem. CDPs don't believe they have much worth or value as a person, so only through interactions with another person (in a codependent relationship) does the CDP have any sense of worth or purpose.

Exaggeration of perceived failure and mistakes. CDPs believe that making one mistake means the CDP is a total failure and unworthy of love. CDPs view mistakes personally; for example, the mistake means the CDP is *a bad person,* not someone who simply made an error.

Looking at this list of traits and then recalling the story at the beginning of this chapter, it is not difficult to connect the dots and realize our client was in a multiple codependent relationship. CDPs are not just those who are linked romantically or sexually; CDPs exist within family structures, churches, places of employment, friendships, etc. It is not uncommon for adults in codependent relationships to come from family structures in which the mother and father are in a codependent relationship or there was a codependent parent-child dynamic.

If you find yourself in a codependent relationship, you are going to face a difficult challenge in becoming your own person. By no means are we saying you must sever ties with the person in question, but if you deem the relationship worth continuing, you might consider counseling or family counseling. A skilled professional who works with these types of relationships can help everyone involved learn how to express thoughts and feelings healthfully and set appropriate boundaries.

Drug use becomes most problematic when you realize your life begins to revolve around drug use. The same can be said for codependent relationships. When you create your entire world to surround one person, your ability to be objective diminishes. Think about how your life was when you were under the influence of substances, and compare this to a codependent relationship. The similarities are much more than coincidence.

The first thing you can do is start to turn the focus on yourself. This is not saying you need to become self-centered and self-absorbed. Rather, this means you need to start paying attention to your own thoughts and feelings and giving your own wants and needs a higher place on the list of priorities. For example, try decreasing your obsessive thoughts about the other person (thinking about the other person in a positive way vs. a negative way), decreasing your fear of being judged (by not judging others), journaling your thoughts and feelings (so they become real), making an inventory of things you would like to do (in order to figure out your wants and needs), enjoying someone for who she is versus looking at her as a "project to fix," and listening to your inner voice when it tells you a want, need, hope, dream, etc.

The next thing to do is realize that you cannot be, and are not, responsible for what other people think and feel. It does not matter what you say, you cannot "make" someone feel sad, angry, hurt, or scared. You cannot reach inside someone and flip on his "angry" switch or her "sad" button. You cannot open someone's head and make him think certain thoughts. Other people make up their own minds, choose their own feelings. Indeed, your words and actions hold weight, and you are responsible for any actions that cause another person harm. But that is a far cry from believing your words will "make" someone think, say, feel, or do something.

You must remember that another codependent person will say or do just about anything to keep you in his or her life. If you make a choice to sever ties with someone who is codependent, expect a tremendous amount of backlash. You might hear harsh words or even be physically attacked. The codependent person will feel abandoned, and you might start to feel guilty and tempted to stay in the situation out of a misplaced sense of duty and obligation. If someone feels upset because you are severing ties, you can say, "I understand this upsets you, but I am doing this for me." You might be called names or even threatened, but don't get sucked into a side argument or get off track. If you need to sever ties, keep the conversation extremely brief and focused, and then be on your way. You might be guilt-tripped, but you have no reason to feel guilty when you are doing what you need to do for your own sustained sobriety.

Finally, remember that your own negative thoughts and feelings will creep up when you are alone. You might feel horrible that you have left a relationship. Sometimes relationships end, and, truthfully, some of them end on a bad note. You are not responsible for how the other person chooses to live his or her life after you sever ties; you are responsible for how you live your own life. In time, you will start to focus more on you, your thoughts, your feelings, your wants, your needs. Again, seeking out support groups and possibly a counselor will help you tremendously in continuing sustained sobriety and increasing your independence.

• • • MARY'S STORY • • •

At age twelve, Mary found her parents' supply of alcohol. Mary's first sip, in her own words, rightfully should have been her last. "I hated how it tasted," she says. Mary said it was a cheap brand of scotch and "it tasted like death." She didn't have another drink until a few weeks later. This time, she drank more. "It still tasted like death, but I wanted to feel like everyone else," she recalls. Mary referred to her parents, an uncle, and an older brother. Mary explained that almost every night she'd see the some or all of them become "loose, relaxed, and having fun." She couldn't understand their "adult jokes" and wanted to be part of the fun. Sneaking back to the liquor cabinet, she took "the first bottle I could grab" and locked herself in her room. She forced alcohol into her system until she felt ready to vomit. Mary said her first time ever being high was a few weeks after her first taste of the adult beverage.

Mary described the euphoric feeling as "being an adult." Mary had never felt like this before, but she immediately enjoyed the sensation. She liked not feeling in complete control and she was laughing at the things she was thinking and saying out loud. In the privacy of her room, she felt the walls spinning and flopped on the bed. She slept soundly and woke up the next morning feeling refreshed and happy. She was confused that her thoughts and feelings were no longer euphoric. Indeed, she didn't even understand why she had been giggling and laughing the previous evening. In retrospect, everything seemed ridiculous, not funny. Mary's confusion didn't stop her from experimenting with alcohol again that very evening.

As time went on, Mary continued to sneak alcohol away from her parents' liquor cabinet and into her system. Mary drank almost every night. She started to drink before she went to school. Eventually, Mary's grades slipped and her attendance dwindled. She told her parents she wasn't feeling well (which was usually true), and when she stayed home, she'd drink. Mary stopped going out with her friends, and eventually she stopped doing her schoolwork. By the age of fifteen, Mary had become a truant and no longer attended school.

Mary's parents were upset with her and protested her decisions and choices. But Mary's parents continued to drink to the point of excess, so at nighttime, when the adults would gather and the adult behaviors commenced, all seemed forgotten. Around this time, just after Mary's fifteenth birthday, her parents discovered Mary had been drinking alcohol. She was the one who told them one evening, when all of the adults were present and drinking together. She reported that initially there was silence, followed by her uncle handing her a beer. "Welcome to the club!" he said, smiling as he gave her the beverage. Without so much as a word of protest from anyone else, especially her parents, Mary drank the beer in almost one gulp. "I hated the taste of it, but it won approval from my family," she says. From that day on, Mary drank with her parents, uncle, and brother almost every night.

Without school, without peers, without social supports, Mary did little else but stay at home and drink every night. Her parents called the school almost every day reporting some ailment or other reason she couldn't attend. Although the school threatened investigations for her ongoing truancy, nothing came of it. At age sixteen, Mary officially dropped out of school. Despite the lack of peer supports, Mary was fine with her "adult life." "I wanted to be with my family, and the only time they ever were together was at night. Now, I was with them and we were all a family," she says.

Mary explained that her family was dysfunctional. Her father worked in a shop every day, sometimes seven days a week. "He was what some call a 'functioning alcoholic.' He drank almost every night, but he'd manage to pull it together and scrape through work every day," Mary says. "He'd come home, and immediately he'd drink. Beer, wine, whiskey, it didn't matter. As long as he drank."

Mary's mother worked part time during the day in a store, "but she was sick half the time, or so she said. How she never was fired remains a mystery. She was plastered from dawn until dusk." Mary's uncle lived with her and her family and he didn't have a job. "I think he had disability payments, but I never could get a straight answer. He always had money for booze," Mary says.

Mary's brother "drank one, maybe two beers a night, but never was a power drinker. He was the most responsible adult in the house. He lived with us until he went away to college after I turned sixteen."

Mary explained that her brother drank to "fit in" with the adults in the household, something Mary recognized herself as doing. She remembers: "I wanted to be one of them. I wanted to be a grown-up. They never encouraged me to do well in school, to have friends, or do anything to be a child. But when I saw them drink with each other, I knew I wanted to be part of that. Alcohol was the glue that held us together. If they couldn't be with me when I needed them, I'd find a way to be with them." Drinking was Mary's solution to having a family.

As Mary continued to age, being with her adult family was all that mattered. Birthdays came and went. Her former classmates graduated high school and moved on to jobs, college, marriage, and careers. Mary continued to live at home. As long as she drank with her family, she was taken care of. Her father continued to work, as did her mother, and with some money from her uncle, she wanted for nothing: room and board plus massive quantities of alcohol. At age twenty-three, Mary was dependent on her mother, father, and uncle to provide for basics. Mary never got a driver's license, never held a job, had no friends, and didn't have any plans for her future.

"I lived in that house, and when I went out, I went with a family member. That was usually a trip to the liquor store," she says.

One night, a few weeks before her twenty-fourth birthday, Mary drank too much. She remembers drinking several shots and then everything going black. Two days later, Mary woke up in a hospital room in critical condition.

"I almost killed myself. Severe alcohol poisoning. My uncle said I just dropped like a stone on the floor and everyone panicked. They called the ambulance and I was admitted to the hospital via the emergency room," Mary says.

The hospital emergency room doctor and social worker contacted a local rehabilitation facility for treatment. At the time, Mary thought, "No way. There's no way I'm going to treatment. I don't have a problem. I just had bad luck." Mary refused to enter treatment because she didn't want to be away from her family.

"Looking back, it was so highly dysfunctional, but they were all I had. I wasn't going to leave all of that. I didn't know how. I was terrified. It never—not once—occurred to me that drinking could or would kill me," she says.

Mary went back home, and the pattern of heavy drinking continued. Less than two months later, Mary was back in the emergency room. Again, she refused treatment. Mary was power drinking and "it was pretty much all day, every day." She went to the emergency room again in another month. And again. And again. After her ninth visit to the emergency room, the doctor told her, "The next time you come here, you won't leave except in a casket." Mary said she didn't care, "because who ever heard of alcohol killing anyone?"

It was fate that heard her question and provided the answer. While Mary was in her ninth stay at the hospital for alcohol poisoning, her parents and uncle came to visit her. They looked grim. Her father sat down next to her and started to cry. Mary says: "I never saw him cry. My mother just stood there looking ashen. My uncle had tears in his eyes, and it was him who told me the news: My brother died earlier that day while away at college."

At the time, Mary didn't know how, but she found out later that evening that it was a drunk driver who hopped a curb and slammed into her brother who was out running. "My brother stopped drinking while he was at school. And he's killed by a drunk driver," Mary says.

In a rare moment of complete sobriety, Mary wept. She hadn't seen her brother in almost two years. "He didn't want to be a part of all of us anymore. I thought he didn't love us, but now I know he had to get away from us so he could be his own person. And a drinker killed him," she says. Mary agreed the next day to enter treatment.

During her time in treatment, Mary argued. She fought. She bickered. She rationalized. She took the victim stance. She blame-shifted. She did and said anything she could in order to minimize her drug usage and attempt to convince others that she didn't have a problem. But other clients and staff reminded her of the tremendous loss she had. Not just of her brother, but of her adolescence and her own life. Mary had been isolated with her family for so long, she didn't even know who the president of the United States was. Mary's education was how to be a power drinker, and alcohol had taken a massive toll on her. Mary said the main spark for her transformation was seeing how much alcohol had taken from her.

"I looked like I was in my early forties instead of almost twenty-five," she says. "I looked like hell. I didn't know I was supposed to look young, and I thought the bags under my eyes, my stringy hair, my dangling skin, were just part of being an adult."

The second thing that pushed Mary into sustained sobriety was what she described as the "sudden flash of insight as to everything I had failed to acquire, and more importantly, what I had lost. I had nothing. I was nothing."

After forty-three days in the program, Mary started to take treatment seriously. She began, with assistance from other clients in the program, to read the materials and work on them. She embraced the fact that she did have a problem with alcohol and that her master, alcohol, had demanded a terrible toll in her ongoing addiction. Mary learned to use the behavioral tools she was being shown in treatment. Her struggle was harder because she had no job and nowhere to live, except back with her alcohol-using and enabling family. She had no social supports, but Mary pushed hard. She made contacts with support groups that came in to the program to speak to clients, and she was able to find sober housing in the community. Mary was set for graduation almost a hundred days after entering the program.

Mary entered sober housing and stayed there for three months. During that time, she was able to secure an identification card, find a part-time job, and start taking driving lessons. Within one year, Mary had a full-time job and an apartment and was working toward her GED. After three years, Mary was a successful applicant to a local college and began taking coursework in public health.

"I never could see how much control drugs and alcohol had over me, my family, everything," she says. "I never knew how much I gave up in order to fit in. I wasn't molested. I wasn't abused. I wasn't degraded. I simply was accepted as 'one of them' because I acted like them. That's all I ever wanted. The price paid for my sobriety was the death of my brother, a most terrible wake-up call. Every day I remind myself, 'I can, I will, I want to.' I lived wrong for years; now I'm living right."

REFLECTION QUESTIONS

- Which relationships in your life are codependent?

_____

_____

_____

- What are the benefits of being alone vs. remaining in an unhealthy relationship?

_____

_____

_____

- What protests do you think you might hear from family or friends?

_____

_____

_____

- How can you counter their complaints or accusations?

  _____

  _____

  _____

CHAPTER FIVE

Battling Boredom

A lot of people, once they are sober, report being bored. This is ironic, because boredom is one of the reasons people list when they start using drugs. The boredom reported has been described as lasting a "painfully long amount of time" and "minutes seem like years." A lot of people can't stand their lives to one degree or another, so they start abusing substances. Boredom serves only to amplify that.

Now, here you are, out of treatment, ready to face the world. You're working on yourself, you're working to build sober supports, you're working to distance yourself from toxic relationships…and you're finding you can't handle the boredom. You have a lot of time on your hands and nothing to do. Much worse, you have almost nobody with whom to pass the time.

Boredom usually starts with some sort of restlessness. You might find it difficult to sit still, read, watch television, or do anything that requires less from you than running at full speed. This restlessness is so intense that there's a strong desire to go full throttle at *something* just to alleviate the overwhelming sense of nothingness happening in your life. What do most people do at this point? They become busy. They engage in all sorts of activities and do as much as possible, all so the boredom won't take hold.

Unfortunately, this has a major drawback.

Think about when someone is grieving, especially when there's a death involved. One of the most common pieces of advice is, "Just get busy and stay busy." Although this might sound helpful, it really tells the person to distract himself instead of dealing with his grief. As long as you stay busy, we reason, you have no time to feel sad. You'll be doing far too much to think about your loss.

This is a deadly trap for people who believe staying busy equals being healthy. Consider someone who goes on vacation because she needs a break from her busy life. She spends a tremendous amount of time planning the trip. She has to hurry home, make reservations for her flight, book a rental car, get a hotel room lined up, plan an itinerary, rush to the airport, rush from one flight to the connecting flight, spend time standing in lines to get her rental car, drive to her hotel, unpack, get a few hours of sleep so she can be up at 5 a.m. to make all of her itinerary stops, rush around to see all the sights, check out of her hotel at the end of her trip, return her rental car, rush to the airplane terminal, rush to the connecting flight back home, and then flop down on her bed exhausted from the vacation *she took to unwind!*

You cannot relax if you are rushing. Similarly, you cannot diminish your grief if you never spend time grieving. Grieving is a natural process and—this might surprise you—it is healthy. Processing your thoughts and feelings, even if you are alone, helps you learn to cope with those feelings of emptiness and sadness. We know grief won't be fixed by ignoring it; you can't substitute a series of behaviors in order to remove a behavioral response.

Think about your sustained sobriety. Regardless of your strong desire to remain sober, you need time to process what it's like to *be* sober. Sobriety means giving up many of the things that used to occupy your time in insobriety. This usually involves severing ties with some people, places, and things. Therefore, as with the death of a loved one, you are in mourning. You grieve the loss of those people, places, and things. You have a void in your life and you want to fill that void. The solution, seemingly, is to get busy and *stay* busy. This is when you usually hear someone say, "Ninety meetings in ninety days." The problem is, even if you attend sober support meetings frequently—and we absolutely encourage you to have sober social support—you are substituting one addictive behavior for another. Attending massive amounts of meetings turns into something that occupies all of your time. Some might argue this is not a bad thing, because you're doing something that helps you stay sober. But the price you pay is that you are wrapped up in attending meetings so much that you don't have time to live your life. Too much of a good thing, after all, is still too much.

Overdoing something, even when it has perceived benefits, is still overdoing it and actually can be counterproductive if not downright harmful. If doing something full-throttle were truly beneficial, most people would be in treatment for a year or two. Counselors know that such a thing as over-treatment exists, and it's harmful and detrimental to the sustained sobriety of their clients. Therefore, there comes a time when it is necessary to make a healthy severance of the clinical relationship and have the client begin her new life.

Boredom, on some level, is a natural part of transitioning into a sober lifestyle and finding new ways to fill your time with activities that amuse, challenge, or entertain you. You should spend your time feeding your soul, not your habit.

You might even choose to spend your time doing something adventurous or taking healthy risks. But some people who have given up drugs become adrenaline junkies, hooked on risky and unsafe activities that "make them feel alive." For many in recovery, that need to "feel alive" is what drew them to using drugs in the first place. Now sober, they replace one unhealthy behavior with another, putting themselves in potential danger just to get a thrill.

The biggest thing to remember about boredom in sobriety is that it won't make you sick or kill you. Boredom doesn't hurt anyone, although it sure can be agonizing. You undoubtedly will feel some sort of anxiety, and it's possible you might feel some level of sadness and depression. These feelings are normal! Remember, you've removed old stimuli, and now you're looking for things to keep you engaged. Not knowing what you're going to do or not knowing what's coming next naturally produces feelings of anxiety and depression.

But in sobriety, you are able to start exploring hobbies and activities with a clear head. You have an entire world open for your exploration. Perhaps you want to learn how to program computers. Maybe you want to watch a television program and understand all of the nuances—while sober. Even something as simple as sitting on a park bench and observing the day go by becomes different when viewed through sober eyes. Considering how many millions of activities and hobbies this world has to offer, it is unreasonable to dismiss *everything* as being dull, uninteresting, or not worthy of your pursuit.

The final thing to keep in mind about your boredom is that this is actually not boredom. Instead of feeling bored, what you're feeling is complete *freedom*. You are free to explore things you wouldn't have or couldn't have while you were high. In your sobriety, you are discovering that you have more time, more capability, and more options. When you were high, you were severely limited in what you could do. Freedom means you can move in and out of activities, sometimes multiple activities every day, without having to spend a significant portion of your time chasing your drug of choice. Even if you long for the so-called "good old days" of being high, think about how much time you *wasted* and how much of your life you *wasted* when you were:

- Hunting down your dealer or finding someplace to buy alcohol;

- Stealing, scamming, or otherwise hustling the money for your next fix or drink;
- Walking, driving, or getting a ride to meet your dealer;
- Making the deal or the purchase;
- Finding a place to get high and/or drunk;
- Getting high or drunk;
- Recovering from getting high or drunk;
- And then repeating the entire cycle.

This was your life as an addict!

So consider: Were you really *alive,* or were you going through the motions?

We encourage you to grieve the loss of your past while welcoming with open arms the new relationship you have with the most important person in your life: you! Once you are able to look at the person in the mirror and start the process of accepting that person, the hardest part of your journey is over.

• • • TRACY'S STORY • • •

Picture a remote rural setting: Small town, a few hundred people, everyone knows everyone else. Life is slow, casual, and leisurely. The hustle and bustle of the big city is only a dream for some, and a nightmare for others. Living here, a day can seem like a lifetime. Many yearn to live in a place like this, but others desire to go somewhere bigger. Tracy had been born in this small town. She knew the city was only a three-hour drive away, but that drive might as well have been infinite. She had no means to visit the city except when her mother wanted to go there for a visit, which was infrequently. Tracy had resigned herself to the fact that she was going to stay in this tiny town forever.

She graduated high school at the top of her class, which had only thirty-eight students. Tracy knew that being "top of her class" meant only so much coming from such a small place. And beyond graduation, she had no hopes, no ambitions, and no drive. She'd never thought about college, and the college recruiters never came to her town. A few military recruiters would show up every now and then, but Tracy didn't want to join. Tracy's only hope was to get a typical job in her typical community and live a typical life. She found a boyfriend, but she didn't really want to be with him in a relationship. Tracy didn't want to work her job. She didn't want to do anything. She wanted out.

Tracy didn't have the means to plan her escape to the city. She had no car, and the small salary she earned as a waitress in the local café was hardly enough to pay her bills. Her boyfriend worked for a local grain company, and together they had enough money left over every month for whatever they wanted. In this small town, having money didn't mean anything if you couldn't spend it. They still didn't have enough to buy a car, but Tracy's boyfriend reasoned that they didn't need one, because they could walk everywhere in their small community.

One day Tracy's boyfriend came home from work and told her he had a plan for their extra money. He knew someone who was a truck driver and the driver offered to cut Tracy's boyfriend in on a deal to start selling small quantities of methamphetamine. For a hundred dollars or so, they could buy and resell for three or four hundred dollars. Her boyfriend rationalized they could start to sell the meth, and with the large amount of extra money, buy a car, and get out of the small town. Many arguments ensued. Tracy had never used drugs, or even seen drugs, and she didn't drink. Eventually, she relented and her boyfriend made the purchase. With some pressure from her boyfriend, Tracy "sampled the product." A long story made short, Tracy and her boyfriend never became the dealers of meth as they had envisioned. Instead, they became hooked on meth and became customers.

Tracy's erratic behavior was noticeable to everyone, and in a short time, she ran afoul of the law. She was given a chance to get clean and was sent to treatment. Tracy resented being in treatment, but at the same time, she looked forward to the experience because it was something new. She told her counselor that she'd used the meth out of boredom. She didn't want to keep experiencing life over and over again on the same bland terms. Therefore, she reasoned, using methamphetamine would take away the dullness of existence and be *something* versus the same old *nothing*.

Meth did indeed "take away" everything and gave her something to do. Emotionally, she'd never felt better. Mentally, she was focused and able to tackle anything.

Meth delivered relief from the dreary, drab life she had lived. She now felt like she was living for the first time.

Tracy continued using meth even when she saw her life falling apart. She no longer went to work. She no longer paid her bills. People from her town are friendly, but everyone knows everyone else's business. So, Tracy and her boyfriend soon were known as the local "meth-heads," and everyone avoided them. People stopped being nice. People stopped helping. Tracy started stealing, and her boyfriend stole a car to drive to the city to get more meth.

Tracy ended up in treatment due to her illegal activities. She's been fighting to stay clean for more than a year since her graduation. As she said, "I started to use because I had no existence. I'm wanting to use again because I'm afraid I'll get bored and start to think about how alive I felt. That rush can't be beat."

Reflection Questions

• What worries you most about feeling bored?

_____

_____

_____

• What are some hobbies, skills, or activities you'd like to try with your newfound free time?

_____

_____

_____

- What parts of you did you let fall away during your period of addiction?

  _____

  _____

  _____

- How can you use your time to get back to the real you?

  _____

  _____

  _____

CHAPTER SIX

Encountering Temptation

Many people realize, on one level or another, that when they leave treatment, they're going to re-enter a world where they're bombarded with things that remind them of the lifestyle they once held dear. Temptation will surround them. It's difficult to walk or drive anywhere in the United States and not see a billboard, sign, or advertisement or hear a radio or television ad for alcohol. Thankfully advertising illegal drugs remains illegal, but many people discover mundane items can stir certain thoughts and feelings. As we discussed in Chapter 1, these things that stir up thoughts and feelings of wanting to use again are often called triggers.

In common parlance, a trigger is any stimulus, event, or condition that can lead to someone abusing substances again. For example, the sight of a beer bottle, the smell of a cigarette, exposure to needles, etc.

One problem with the notion of triggers is that they're presumed to be absolute. In other words, once a trigger, always a trigger. Therefore, people warn and threaten you that if you don't avoid exposure to triggers, you'll relapse!

No evidence exists whatsoever that so-called triggers exist. As a matter of fact, at ARC, we don't call them triggers.

We instead refer to them as excuses. Take a beer bottle, for example. A beer bottle has absolutely *zero* influence over you. It cannot make you drink. It cannot do anything to you.

We do not agree with the notion of so-called triggers, because once you believe something is a trigger, you give that thing *power and control* over your life. You voluntarily are telling that thing: "You control my thoughts and my feelings. You own me, and I submit to you." We are convinced that people do not want mundane objects such as a beer bottle, a needle, a cotton ball, steel wool, tissue paper, hair ties, etc., to hold such sway over them. Despite that, so many people are convinced that they are surrounded by these so-called triggers that life becomes terrifying. These people are afraid to engage in activities because they will be surrounded by their triggers. They think they'll be tempted to use and will go back to using.

Removing the power from these triggers and identifying them for what they really are—*excuses*—empowers you. If you see a beer bottle, you see a beer bottle. Otherwise, you might never leave your house. Think about the myriad things that are associated with drinking alcohol: the bar where you used to drink; the smell of a cigarette; neon signs; someone named Fred (because he was your bartender); brown coasters (they were used for your beer at your favorite bar); mahogany (the type of wood your favorite bar was made from); four-legged barstools. The list goes on!

At this point, you're probably thinking, "Gee, that's a lot of triggers." Exactly. You can see how the excuses can pile up and how you might be tempted to start avoiding living life. Instead, you live based on a fear reaction instead of a thought response. You become afraid to do this or do that because of what you *might* encounter. You also, if you buy into these excuses, are saying you do not believe in yourself and you do not trust yourself to maintain the strength you have.

In the ARC program, we run an exercise every three or four months in which we ask every client to come to the whiteboard and write down his or her so-called triggers. We see the usual suspected triggers, and then the board starts to fill with what we consider absolutely absurd triggers. We spend time dissecting these and explain that the client will never be able to re-enter society and never be able to go outside his or her room because *everything* is a trigger. *Everywhere* he goes will be a trigger. The client will have to live in a sterile bubble, ostracized from society, to avoid succumbing to temptation due to *all of these triggers*!

Clients then start to understand the sheer absurdity of the huge list on the whiteboard. They start to understand that these things have no power. The power is in the client to use or not to use. The client comes to understand that if he or she accepts the existence and power of triggers, this is enabling. If the client comes to understand the power remains completely with the client, this is empowerment.

Consider how trigger excuses might keep you from living your life. Will you keep yourself away from events such as barbeques, holiday gatherings, and social outings out of fear? We recognize that the fear of using again is real. But *you* own your fears and strengths. We believe being cautious, observant, and vigilant is appropriate when you are in sustained sobriety. We believe knowing what *could* trip you up is valuable information to keep in mind. We also believe you need to live your life and enjoy the life you have. Going to a barbeque might be difficult, but there are many other things to do at a barbeque besides drinking or using drugs. You can go bowling without drinking beer. You can visit old friends, and, if they insist on using drugs, *you can always leave!* Remember, for every excuse you create as to why you'll use again, you can list at least ten reasons why you will *not* use. The strength is within you to make the right choice.

Some clients come to believe that in time, they'll be able to use alcohol or drugs again. Some clients think they have their problems licked, all is well, and there's no need for further exploration of the tools offered in treatment. The belief that treatment has "cured" the client comes up from time to time. When we hear about that, we almost inevitably hear that the client is contemplating using drugs again just to see if she truly has beaten the addiction.

The question remains: Can I have just *one* drink or *one* hit of my favorite drug after treatment and not get addicted again? The answer is simply, "Maybe." You also can be bitten by a poisonous snake and there's a slim chance you'll survive, but it's doubtful you'll take your chances with the poisonous snake. There's also a slim chance that you can enter a casino, bet $1, and win the multimillion-dollar jackpot in one pull of a slot machine. But it's doubtful that you'll be able to do such a thing. In other words, though it's certainly *possible* you can start using alcohol and drugs with getting addicted again, the odds are severely against you—if not totally against you.

There's a myth called the "Gambler's Fallacy" in which a person believes that if something happens for a long time, the opposite is bound to happen: *"I'm due for a change of luck!"* A tremendously high number of people leaving treatment believe that because they have been "down on their luck" for so long and their addiction was so severe, they are now bound to stay sober. Some people believe that, even as they ingest addictive substances, they stand only a slim chance of becoming addicted again because they are "due" for a long period of sustained sobriety. *And they think this while they are actively abusing substances!*

The fallacy, of course, has no bearing in reality. There is zero evidence that things will "turn a corner" just because something has been a certain way for so long. The Gambler's Fallacy remains a trap because the person doesn't do anything to change his behavior; he simply believes that luck or fate will kick in and things will start to swing in a new direction. Think about that for a moment and ask yourself, does going to treatment guarantee a change of luck or a shift in direction? And does leaving treatment mean you can start to abuse substances again and somehow be protected from the addictive properties of those substances?

Too many people believe that changing their thinking protects them from getting high. If only things were that simple!

We absolutely believe that someone can drink alcohol and *not* become addicted to it if that person's drug of choice is opiates, cocaine, methamphetamine, etc. Cross-drug addiction is not supported by medical science, and no studies conclusively demonstrate that one drug addiction equals addiction to every drug. There is no scientific support for the 1950s mentality that you cannot, under any circumstance, use *any* sort of addictive substance once you are in addiction or recovering from addiction. If cross-addiction were a real thing, every single thing on the planet that has an addictive property would be addictive to an addict! Therefore, yes, it's possible that you *can* pick up a beer and safely drink it if alcohol is not your drug of choice.

However…

We ask these questions: What would prompt you to think you need to use another substance instead of your drug of choice? Why are you looking for an excuse to do another drug instead of your drug of choice? What part of you is saying, "Give up heroin, but start drinking," or, "Don't pick up that beer; do cocaine instead." When you are actively looking to replace your drug of choice with another, you are engaging in substitutionary behavior. You're looking to use something that will give you some sort of high or stimulation that might resemble the effects you used to get on your drug of choice.

This is highly dangerous.

If you find yourself needing to pick up another drug, then you should understand that you're still addicted—to the need to put something in your body to feel "different." If you're wanting to pick up a beer instead of a needle, or snort a powder instead of smoking a rock, we strongly encourage you to seek psychiatric care, because you might have an imbalance of certain chemicals in your brain. Years of drug or alcohol abuse can deplete or otherwise alter some things in your body and brain that might require certain psychiatric medications. These medications can help stabilize some or all of the imbalance. The need to pick up that beer or smoke that joint (even with another drug being your drug of choice) is the desire to self-medicate and make things "feel" right. Psychiatric assistance might help you best.

Therefore, our strong advice to you is *not* to tempt yourself. Avoid the desire to jump back into using substances, even if you have convinced yourself you'll never get addicted to something new. Remember what you thought before treatment? You thought, "I'll never get addicted to this. I have it under control. I control it; it doesn't control me." By now, haven't those thoughts come and gone?

The odds are strongly stacked against you if you decide you can start using another substance, and we believe any need to use illicit substances speaks to the core issues that led you to start abusing substances in the first place.

What if you're headed down that path? What if you're feeling those old feelings and old thoughts about using again? What if the pull is too powerful to resist? What if those old people, places, and things are too overwhelmingly strong to ignore? Are you going to use again? Are you going to relapse?

You might even be asking yourself, "Am I going to fail… again?"

• • • RICH'S STORY • • •

Rich had a great job. At forty-five years old, he was seen as one of the most successful salespeople in his region. Rich was popular when he would show up at the cigar bar. He bought drinks for people and would sit and talk with anyone and everyone. As soon as he pulled up in his brand new convertible, everyone knew Rich was in the house and it was time to cut loose. The waitresses and bartenders knew they were going to be tipped big-time.

But once Rich left the bar, he went home to a huge, empty house, where he would trudge around until he flopped on the couch or his bed. At one time, Rich's house had been a home, but now, Rich was divorced. His wife and children had moved out long ago.

It was no secret that Rich had been a "power drinker"

since his high school days. He was lucky and managed to get through school with barely passing grades. Rich had been popular in school, and he quickly found a job and became a top salesman in his firm. Rich already was living under the "good ol' boy" mentality—every salesperson he knew was a power drinker. Rich's father had been a salesman, and Rich couldn't recall a memory in which his father didn't have an alcoholic beverage in his hands. So Rich continued two traditions: being a great salesman and being a power drinker. He also vehemently denied that alcohol had ever been a problem.

Rich's wife and closest friends disagreed with his assessment. They knew Rich when he was sober and when he was "just cutting loose." Rich said he drank to help cut the pressure of his job, which, admittedly, was stressful but extremely lucrative. Rich could afford all sorts of luxuries, and in his worldview, as long as he made money, he had no problems. Despite protests from her parents, Rich's ex-wife had married him when they were young. She had thought she could save Rich from himself. After eight years, two children, and many nights of Rich's black-out anger, passing out behind the wheel of the car, and otherwise outrageously unacceptable behaviors, she took the children and left, filing for divorce the next day.

A year after the divorce, Rich continued to come home to the same huge, empty house. He drank a large quantity of alcohol before the divorce (which, according to him, was the result of his wife being "an ungrateful bitch"), but since the split, he had been drinking more than anyone else even realized. He had been pulled over at least four times in two years for drinking and driving, but he'd never been arrested. Rich couldn't even remember how he got home most nights; his life consisted of working and drinking.

Rich's supervisor at work noted that Rich's behavior had slumped. Although Rich had always been a drinker, in the past year, Rich had started to show changes that were disturbing. He came into work late, or sometimes not at all. When he was at work, he would miss sharing or taking down important information. When at meetings with staff or clients, he would appear to "nod off" or come to the meetings disheveled. Rich brushed off all of these things as "being tired" or "distracted," but his supervisor recognized what was happening and gave Rich a choice: Get into treatment or get a new job.

Rich chose to enter treatment, where he initially played out the "it's not the alcohol, it's everyone else" series of excuses. Rich blame-shifted, took the victim stance, rationalized, justified, and portrayed himself to be an upstanding guy who every now and then "had an extra drink." Rich's drinking was not a problem, according to Rich. When it was pointed out that Rich had no real friends, just drinking buddies; his wife and children had left him, and they hadn't been in touch in almost one year; and his boss had sent him to treatment to get help, Rich stormed out of treatment. He walked down the street, found the first bar he could, and drank himself into a stupor.

Rich detoxed and re-entered treatment two days later. Despite Rich's behavior—turning to alcohol when things got tough or stressful—he denied he had a problem. He blamed the counselors, the administrators, and the other clients for his recent alcohol-fueled binge. He even blamed the bartender, stating, "He should have known I wasn't well. I just walked out of treatment, but he served me anyway." Rich was deep in his excuses and justifications, but he was a life worth saving.

It took some time, but with the work of other clients and the staff, Rich started to see he had a problem. But Rich was concerned, because all he knew was drinking. As a salesperson, every lunch, every dinner, every meeting, every social conference was an alcohol-fueled gathering. If you weren't drinking, you weren't considered "cool" or "one of the guys." Rich knew that if he stopped drinking, he might not be accepted the same as he had been. Rich was terrified that everything he knew would be taken from him if he stopped. Therefore, Rich had reservations about cutting alcohol out of his life entirely. Rich also knew that he wasn't one of the ones who could drink in moderation. Rich said, "I could stop drinking, sure, but I know that one drink is all it will take and I'm gone." Rich had no will power to moderate his drinking. Therefore, for Rich, the solution was total abstinence.

Rich persevered and graduated four months later, but he was nervous about returning to work. He was nervous that he would be pressured and would give in to alcohol.

He enrolled in aftercare and managed to stay sober for a few months, but he stopped coming to his sessions. When we did reach him, we knew he was drunk. Slurring his speech, he said he'd gone to a conference, become scared, and started to drink. We asked him what had scared him, and he said, "I was scared I wasn't going to be the same guy I've always been."

Rich sobered up and re-admitted himself to aftercare. He stayed enrolled and managed to stay sober despite tremendous pressure to do otherwise. In his last phone call to us, Rich said, "I'm fighting my demons every day. This is hard—way harder than I ever imagined. But instead of me worrying about demons, I'm blessed by the visits of the angels."

Rich's children had started to visit him again, and he mentioned the possibility of reconciliation with his wife.

REFLECTION QUESTIONS

- What do you think would happen if you started using a different substance than you've used in the past?

_____

_____

_____

- What seems appealing about that? What are the risks?

_____

_____

_____

- How do you feel when you know you've made a healthy, if difficult, choice?

  _____

  _____

  _____

  _____

CHAPTER SEVEN

Common Questions and Thinking Errors

Going to treatment doesn't make you sober any more than going to a garage makes you a car. By now, we hope you realize that treatment doesn't "fix" or "cure" you. To be sure, there's no such thing as a cure for substance abuse.

That sounds terribly demoralizing. But lack of a cure does not mean it'll get worse.

Substance abuse is a disorder that doesn't go away. It might diminish tremendously over time, but the underlying behaviors that led to your substance abuse will remain unless you are seeking treatment to work on those behaviors. Even with treatment to work on the behaviors that led to your substance abuse, seeds of those behaviors linger. Sometimes those seeds grow back into the same maladaptive behaviors we worked so hard to remove.

Keep in mind that substance abuse is a diagnosis that exists within the field of mental health. Substance abuse is a behavioral disorder, and most behavioral disorders are not curable. They are, however, *treatable*. This means that with active treatment, the signs and symptoms can be diminished or possibly eliminated. The key word is *active*. If you are working *actively* to decrease, diminish, minimize, or remove the problem behaviors, you stand a high chance of maintaining sustained sobriety.

"Don't I Have a Disease? Aren't Diseases Curable?"

At ARC, we do not subscribe to the disease model of addiction. Most programs believe that substance abuse is a medical disease. You might hear addiction called a "brain disease." Tremendous amounts of scientific and medical research conclusively demonstrate that there is no causal link genetically or related to brain structure and addiction. Even if addiction *could* be considered a disease, the strong behavioral component of substance abuse is not disputed by proponents of the disease model of addiction.

The good news is, behavioral diagnoses such as substance abuse have high rates of successful outcomes. Additionally, even though substance abuse is a behavioral issue, this does not mean you must neglect or ignore medical input regarding your substance abuse. For example, if you have a problem with opiate abuse, it might benefit you to seek medical advice and possibly prescriptions such as methadone, Suboxone, or Vivitrol. These medications will help reduce symptoms of opiate withdrawal. They absolutely will not cure you, but they will help make life bearable by reducing physical discomfort and allowing you to focus mentally. Also, you might have co-existing medical conditions that can negatively affect your progress toward sustained sobriety. Therefore, you need to have ongoing, co-occurring medical supervision and possibly treatment as you work toward sobriety. We wholeheartedly encourage you to seek medical consultation for *any* substance abuse issue, and we also encourage you to enroll in counseling to help reduce or remove the behaviors that led to the substance abuse.

"I'm Worried that I'm Going to Be a Failure!"

You might have heard from various individuals that "relapse is part of recovery." You even might have heard people insist that you are destined to abuse substances again and there's nothing you can do about it. Some people will tell you relapse and recovery are cyclical and neverending. These doom-sayers will fill you with fear and trepidation. These same people take their own experience and project that onto you and everyone else who uses substances. These people have fallen victim to a fallacy: black-or-white thinking. These people believe that you will either be completely successful or completely fail. Because ongoing sobriety is seen as a complete success, any insobriety is viewed as complete failure. They say that if you have ever abused substances, you have completely failed and will continue to do so. After all, *they* failed and *you* will, too.

The truth is that abusing substances is not a failure. And even if you choose to believe that abusing substances is a sort of failure, the failure is temporary, not permanent. A failure retains the capability to be remedied. Thus, if you have made an error, the error can be corrected. If you break your arm, are you a failure? If you come down with the flu, are you a failure? If you wear the wrong shirt to work, are you a failure? At what point does the failure stop being failure and become a mistake or an oversight or a slip? When does a relapse become a recovery? When does recovery become *recovered*?

Like the disease model of addiction, the 1950s mentality believes, "once an addict, always an addict." There is a great deal of talk that you are always in recovery and you must constantly fight and claw your way to sobriety. Every waking moment, according to those who think you'll always be in recovery, must be spent actively engaging in sobriety and avoiding any and all people, places, and things that could remotely tempt you…*because you will fail*!

The scientific and clinical evidence do not support the notion of "once an addict, always an addict." Vast quantities of peer-reviewed, evidence-based research demonstrate that those who once held an addiction do not necessarily carry that addiction long-term.

To reiterate, failure is not guaranteed! Failure is *not* what happens if you get out of treatment and use or abuse substances. You might use again, but that indicates your coping skills weren't strong enough. And, because there is no "cure" for addiction, it's impossible to "fail" by using again. If you believe addiction is a disease, then ask yourself if a cancer patient "fails" because his cancer comes back after it was in remission.

The proponents of the disease model of addiction believe that the person who has the so-called disease isn't truly responsible for her problem; it's not the *drugs*, it's the *disease*. The person abusing substances is simply reacting to her *disease*—it's not about behaviors. The problem with this outdated method of thinking is that this enables the substance abuser by turning the substance abuser into a victim of circumstance. Empowerment is completely removed. Continuing with the previous example, a person who has a disease might not be able to control signs and symptoms of his disease. A person with cancer might come out of remission through no action of his own. A person who has a problem with alcohol can take steps to not drink alcohol. Without alcohol, the so-called disease of alcoholism vanishes! The same is *not* true of any real disease.

Because we know substance abuse is not a disease and instead is a behavioral issue, we do not blame your genetics, your brain structure, or anything biological.

"Am I Going to Relapse?"

We do not accept the notion of "relapse." The word *relapse* has the notion of failure built into it. If you believe that you will relapse, you accept that failure is destined. As already discussed, failure is neither an accurate nor honest way to perceive life after treatment. However, if you accept the notion of relapse, you accept the notion of failure and you accept that you are not going to remain sober.

Instead of "relapsing" or "failing," we call this "being human." We know, for example, we shouldn't eat fast food when we are trying to lose weight, but we might do it anyway. We also know we shouldn't have another drink, but we do. We know we shouldn't have that rock of crack cocaine, but we do. Giving in to our temptations simply reaffirms our humanity. This does not mean you must go out and indulge in the things you are hoping to avoid. Quite the opposite! But if you do indulge, you're not being bad, evil, immoral, a failure, relapsing, etc. You're telling the world, "I'm a person and I'm fighting tons of impulses, thoughts, feelings, and this struggle is difficult!"

Now, that previous paragraph will give some people an excuse to abuse substances again and then say, "Hey, I'm only human." Those who do so are making excuses and rationalizing; they're justifying and minimizing their behaviors. It is quite a different thing to *struggle* versus to have excuses lined up when you do use. Some people aren't ready to give up using drugs, and we call that "having reservations." This means you say you want to stop, but in reality, the desire remains and so do the excuses.

Even when we are completely admitting our humanity and admitting that we sometimes give in to our emotions vs. our reason, we still are coming up short. Therefore, we have to buckle down, do our own emotional inventory homework, figure out why we're drawn to doing the things we know aren't in our best interests, and work on a solid plan to stay on the straight and narrow. You might have heard the expression, "The struggle is real." We agree, and when we struggle, we feel *real!* As much as the struggle can create powerful feelings of all sorts, it also can create the potential for us to rise up, overcome, and tackle the challenges in front of us. We can give in to our passions, making those excuses along the way to become a rationalizer, justifier, blame-shifter, etc., or we can master our passions and become the conqueror. We think being a conqueror sounds a lot better than taking the victim stance!

"But If It's Behavioral, Then Addiction Is My Fault!"

Sure, addiction is behavioral. We do not argue that.

But there's no need to find fault or place blame.

The driving question every person who abuses drugs wants to know is, "Why do I do this?" The answer is, "We're not 100 percent sure." You might never understand exactly why you abuse substances, and you might need to make your peace with that. But you absolutely can discover behavioral solutions to minimize or eliminate the desire to abuse substances. Therefore, if your substance abuse is behavioral in origin, you can learn to change or eliminate those learned behaviors that led to your substance abuse. In short, if you learned it, you can change or unlearn it!

Any learned behavior can be changed, re-directed, or unlearned. Once you accept this (and remember, addiction is learned, not innate!), you empower yourself. The belief and knowledge that you can and will change your behavior is liberating. You have the ability and power to change.

Accepting that you have a disease and that your addiction is genetic and outside of your scope of power to change is *enabling* and gives you a constant source of excuses to keep abusing substances. You accept that it's not your fault (yet you are told you have responsibility for substance abuse), and you cannot control it (yet you are told that you need to change your thinking). That leads you down a path of learned helplessness, not a path of liberation. The former path teaches you to accept your fate and recognize how utterly *powerless* you are; the latter teaches you that you control your fate and have tremendous amounts of power to overcome your substance abuse.

In the end, you will make a choice as to which path leads to sobriety.

Finally, keep in mind that you will never have all of the answers. You need, as stated earlier, a great support system along with competent and informed medical care and excellent aftercare. Combine those with the tools you learned in treatment, and your rate of sustained sobriety skyrockets into the stratosphere! Even then, you still will not have all of the answers. Take comfort in the fact that no one on the planet has all the answers about *anything*. All of us are on a constant quest for knowledge, be it regarding the universe, the oceans, or who is the next reality television star. Our thirst to know more drives us to keep exploring. You are an excellent topic for study and your own personal research. Imagine what you will know about yourself tomorrow that you didn't know today.

For thirty-two years, Edith wavered in and out of a semblance of a life. She had high hopes when she was a child to become a doctor. When she was little, she fell from a tree and broke her arm. The doctor was kind and gave her candy when she was done. She had to wear a cast for many weeks, and when she was ready to have the cast removed, she was excited to see the doctor again. After removal of her cast, he again gave her candy. "I want to be a doctor just like you!" she said when she left. She gave the doctor a hug, and for many years, she thought many times about how much she wanted to be a doctor to help people. Edith loved the idea of helping people. She wanted to be a helper.

But no one told Edith she would need to do well in school. Good grades are essential for entering college and then medical school. Edith was an average student, and when she started high school, her grades slipped into substandard. She had some encouragement from her father, but her mother told her repeatedly, "You're a poor student. You'll never be a doctor." Undaunted, Edith pushed herself to raise her grade-point average, but by the time she was a junior, she was earning Cs. In her free time, Edith pored over medical books from her school library. She didn't understand a lot of what she read. She asked questions of her biology teacher. Still, even after all of her extracurricular studying, Edith's grades did not improve. "See?" her mother asked her, "You can't do it."

Edith's mother, Denise, married for money. Denise was a socialite and well-regarded by her husband's peers. Denise did not want children but had one anyway because it was expected of her. Denise was absent for long stretches of time, sometimes weeks on end, and Edith's father, Jim, was the primary caregiver. Jim did not push back against his wife's drinking. It's fair to say that Denise was the dominant partner in the relationship, although it was Jim's busy but substantial career, Jim's family, and Jim's money that helped put Denise into the high social circles she craved. Denise was superficially charming and glib, but she was an absentee parent.

Denise spent a lot of her time drinking, and Edith witnessed firsthand the terrible effects of alcohol on her mother. Denise would fly into rages for no reason, break down crying over a minor issue, and sometimes not react in the least. Denise did not encourage Edith in any way, and more of Edith's birthdays were spent alone with the housekeeper or her father, when Jim was able to get away from the pressures of his career. Denise belittled her daughter and made sure Edith knew that she, Edith, was nothing. Denise was once heard by the housekeeper calling Edith "a useless pile of flesh" and saying, "If you die, you'll do me a favor. Everyone will come to your funeral." Edith never understood why her mother didn't love her. Maybe the kind doctor who took care of her when she broke her arm was the reason Edith wanted to become a doctor. Edith had received so very little kindness in her life that, when someone expressed it to her, she gravitated toward it.

Edith longed for affection closer to home. She could not find love from the mother who never wanted her, and her father was almost never home. Edith's grades were enough for her to maintain good academic standing, but they were not college material. Edith started to believe what she had been told by her mother for all of her life: She would never amount to anything. Edith stopped caring about her grades. She stopped caring about her appearance. She stopped caring about anything that remotely held her interest. That's when a certain group from her school took notice of Edith.

This group welcomed Edith with open arms. They wanted her to be a part of their clique. For the first time in her life, she felt accepted, wanted, even needed. This group asked her to hang out with them, but they also asked her if she'd be able to help them secure alcohol. Edith knew her mother's bar was fully stocked. Edith would invite some of the group members over after school, or, at times, they'd all skip school and hang out at Edith's house, drinking. Edith's popularity with this fringe group grew, and in time, she became a sort of leader of the group of outcasts. As long as Edith was able to supply alcohol, she had the power. In time, Edith started to steal money from her mother's purse and her father's wallet. Before the middle of her senior year, Edith had stopped going to school altogether and instead proclaimed herself to be the "Queen of the Ball," fancying herself to be a sort of hero-princess to her fellow miscreants. At the same time she dropped out of school, Edith was consuming between six to twelve beers per day, plus assorted liquor.

Edith never graduated from high school. Her mother couldn't have cared less about the welfare of her daughter; after all, by that time, Edith was eighteen years old and no longer mandated to attend school. With Edith a legal adult, Denise could ignore requests to show up for a parent-teacher conference. Edith's father cared, but his career took him all over the globe. He simply could not afford to spend time on his daughter's welfare and education. His only thought was to allow Edith to remain living at home, which he believed would help her get on the right path. He even secured a job for Edith in his company. Edith never showed up for her first day of work. She spent her days and nights at wild parties, drinking alone, or doing absolutely nothing.

Edith never took driver's education. She had learned how to drive a car but could not do so legally. Because Edith was usually under the influence of alcohol, her peers thought it was a good thing she didn't have a license. One of them commented, "You're always so messed up that you couldn't drive straight if you were sober." Edith disregarded her lack of formal driver's education and not having a license regularly. She would often take one of her parents' vehicles, drive to the liquor store with stolen money and a fake ID and purchase alcohol for the party of the day. This was a daily occurrence, and this particular Thursday was no different than the last.

Edith purchased several quarts of alcohol and a few cases of beer, headed over to her friends' apartment, and got the party going. Edith drank around thirteen beers and had ingested several shots of liquor. She remembers blacking out several times that evening, and after her fifth or sixth blackout, she decided to call it a night. A couple people at the party told her to crash there for the night, but Edith said she wanted to sleep in her own bed. One person took Edith's car keys from her, resulting in a brief physical altercation. Edith angrily grabbed the car keys, entered her car, started it, put it in reverse, and backed out of the driveway. Edith doesn't remember anything after her friend took her car keys from her, but she remembers waking up in a hospital room with several tubes plugged into her body. It was daylight outside. Before she blacked out again, Edith remembers screaming and seeing several nurses and a doctor enter her room.

The second time she awoke, it was dark outside. This time, Edith didn't scream. She was scared, but she had no recollection of how she got there and, more important, why she was there. Edith paged the nurse and asked what happened. The nurse took Edith's hand and said she would be back in a few minutes with the social worker. True to her word, within a few minutes, an elderly lady with a kind face entered Edith's room. She introduced herself as Kate. Edith asked what happened. Kate asked Edith if she remembered anything at all. Edith could not recall details. For the next half-hour, Kate spent time talking with Edith in order to see what she remembered. Around that time, a doctor walked in. He was young and didn't say much. Edith asked the doctor what happened. The doctor and social worker exchanged looks. The doctor said: "You had an accident. Try to relax." Edith asked if she was all right. The doctor said that Edith had severe alcohol poisoning and was near death when she came in to the hospital. Edith was confused; she didn't recall any of this. The doctor then said, "There's more, but you'll have to talk with a detective."

"A detective?" Edith asked. The doctor nodded his head. Edith's pulse and blood pressure escalated. She felt sick to her stomach. She knew something was wrong. As if on cue, an older man walked into the room. He looked stern but talked kindly. He introduced himself as Detective Sams. He asked Edith the same questions the social worker and doctor had. Edith repeatedly said she didn't remember anything. Edith was scared, but she wanted answers. She raised her voice and screamed, "Tell me what happened!" Detective Sams said in a calm but forceful voice, "We believe you are responsible for killing someone."

Edith started to cry uncontrollably. She couldn't stop sobbing. She managed to get one word out: "How?" Detective Sams said, "When you started to leave, Sasha tried to stop you. She banged on your window, but you wouldn't stop. She walked behind your car to get you to stop. You hit the gas pedal and ran her over. Edith, Sasha's dead."

Edith started to scream, and she attempted to get out of her bed. The doctor called in a nurse and gave Edith a shot of something. After a few moments, the detective and social worker left the room. The nurse stayed behind for a few more moments, and Edith passed out for several hours.

In the next few days, Edith learned the truth about the events that night. Several witnesses saw her enter her car and accelerate in reverse, backing over Sasha and killing her. Edith's car continued into the street and into a tree; Edith passed out at the steering wheel. At the age of nineteen, Edith's life appeared to be over. She was facing vehicular homicide and several other criminal charges. Additionally, she was recovering from acute alcohol poisoning, malnutrition, and severe dehydration. She remained in the hospital for several days.

During this time in the hospital, no one came to see her. Not her father. Not her mother. Not her "friends." The only one who saw her regularly was Kate, the social worker. Although Edith called her home several times per day and attempted to contact her father, who was out of the country, she never received an answer. Edith was terrified and alone and she didn't know what to do. She only knew she did not want to live her life like this.

It was a tough year for Edith. After she came home from the hospital, her mother would not speak to her except to say, "I told you, you'd never amount to anything. Well, except now you're a murderer." Edith had nowhere to go, so she lived in the poisonous household. Edith's father was still traveling. He offered no support except brief phone calls and a powerful, expensive attorney. Edith was terrified and did not know what to do. Her attorney talked with her but only about her case. He had no advice for her except to "get clean, get sober, and stay out of trouble." Edith remembered the kind doctor from all those years ago. She also remembered the smiling and helpful social worker.

Edith returned to the hospital to speak with Kate.

Kate spent an hour talking with Edith. Kate provided Edith with several phone numbers for rehabilitation facilities and halfway houses. Kate explained that Edith had a problem with alcohol, and although she had been drinking heavily for a few years, she would be able to turn it around if she wanted to. Kate offered to refer Edith to several rehabilitation facilities. Edith accepted Kate's assistance, and after a few phone calls, Edith checked herself into a rehabilitation in-patient program less than thirty minutes from her house.

Edith struggled in treatment because of the legal issues hanging over her head. Additionally, Edith was haunted by the fact that she had killed someone. Edith truly felt remorse for her actions and took responsibility for them.

Edith did not run from what she had done, but she wished she could hide. One day during a break in the group schedule, two police officers came to the treatment center. They were there to arrest Edith. Edith knew why they were there and turned herself over to them. Although Edith was taking responsibility to enter sustained sobriety, she wanted to be accountable for what she had done.

It was discovered that Sasha, the young lady who was killed, was intoxicated and partially to blame for being directly behind the car. Edith faced charges of vehicular homicide, driving without a license, driving while under the influence, and grand theft auto. In the end, due to Edith's willingness to admit culpability and other mitigating circumstances, the judge sentenced Edith to two years in prison. The judge gave Edith some hope: successfully complete rehabilitation, stay clean and sober for five years, and report on felony probation. And after that five-year period, it might be possible to expunge Edith's criminal record. Edith accepted and returned to treatment.

Edith's next several months in treatment were tough. She wrestled constantly with the death of Sasha, her out-of-control drinking, having a felony conviction, and not receiving visitors, phone calls, or letters. No one supported Edith. No one seemed to care.

Except one person.

Kate would check in from time to time. Kate was the only person from the outside who supported Edith. Edith learned in time through her counseling inside of treatment that she had value. She was worthy of love and was capable of giving love. Edith rediscovered her passion. She wanted to help others. She knew she could help people turn their lives around because she was turning her life around. Edith attended Twelve-Step meetings, had a sponsor who truly looked out for her, met weekly with her therapist, and attended several groups in addition to group therapy. Six months after entering treatment, Edith was poised to graduate. Edith's mother did not come to the graduation. Edith's father did not come to the graduation. No one from the outside came to the graduation.

Except one person.

Kate showed up at graduation to encourage Edith and let her know that you can't pick and choose who will support you in life so you need to accept help from wherever it may come. Edith was grateful to have one support in the community who never judged her, never mocked her, never turned her back. Someone was helping Edith. And Edith had always wanted to be a helper. She had forgotten that feeling from so long ago.

Edith had lined up sober living after her graduation. She transitioned to the new housing, found a part-time job, and enrolled in school. Edith completed the GED program and started taking classes at a community college. Edith managed to earn a 3.7 grade-point average and make the Dean's List. Edith's grades were good enough to earn her a scholarship that she used to transfer to a four-year college. Edith had thought about being a doctor, but now she had a different career path in mind: Edith wanted to be a social worker.

Sixteen years later, Edith is a lead clinician at a local hospital helping patients with trauma find their way. Edith is a respected professional whose passion encourages her coworkers and patients.

After all, Edith loves to help people. She always wanted to be a helper.

REFLECTION QUESTIONS

- Based on what you just read in this chapter, has your view on the roots of addiction changed?

  _____

  _____

  _____

- What comes to mind when you hear the word *relapse*?

  _____

  _____

  _____

- Do you believe you will use again? What encourages you to believe you can stay sober?

  _____

  _____

  _____

Tying It All Together

By now, you've probably come to the conclusion that sustained sobriety is challenging. This is because insobriety has really mucked things up for you. You've put in a lot of work thus far, and you'll continue to put in even more work. It won't ever end, but it will become easier. You have proven you have the strength to stop using your drug(s) of choice, and if you had an instance or instances or re-using illicit substances, you've had the presence of mind to stop again and attempt to right yourself.

You know you're going to run into things that tempt you. You inevitably will encounter old places, old people, and old things, because you're living your life. You might experience anxiety, depression, racing thoughts, cold sweats, and other unpleasant sensations. You'll feel feelings and think thoughts that could lead you back down the path of abusing substances. You might encounter people who will encourage you to use with them, or you might run into a situation that reminds you of the perceived good times you had when you were using.

You'll find there are times when you are alone. You won't be able to reach anyone to talk to when you want to use.

You will find times when you can't get to a support meeting, or the meeting will not be productive for you. You will talk with people you think might be helpful, and you'll walk away feeling frustrated and believing no one understands.

There will be times when you feel rundown or sick. You'll be tempted to call or text someone to bring you something to help you out, a little "something to tide you over" until you're back on your feet. You'll have those days and weeks when you are exhausted and just want to say, "Screw it!" and go back to what is familiar, because there's security and safety in what's familiar.

None of this is uncommon. You are not alone. You are not unique in these experiences. You are not the only one who hits hard times, difficult times, seemingly impossible times. Your sustained sobriety—or, more aptly stated, your journey through sustained sobriety—is totally yours. You will experience common situations, but the journey will be yours.

These statements and caveats might sound intimidating, but we share them with you because your best chance of staying true to your path is to understand the potential detours along that path.

This entire book, in addition to your time spent in treatment learning tools for sustained sobriety, prepares you for the encounters you'll have along your journey. The key word is *prepares*. What was learned in treatment and what you retain from this book are meant to enlighten you about what's ahead and give you resources to deal with those issues should they arise. Some people will never have any of these issues come up; some people will have *all* of these issues come up. The majority of people will have some issues from here and there, in no particular pattern. You do not know what problems you'll encounter, if any at all, or when, how often, etc.

If that uncertainty frightens or upsets you, consider: *Everyone's* future is unknown. Even if you were not in recovery from a substance abuse issue, your future would be in flux based on your decisions as well as the decisions of everyone else, including those close to you and people you'll never even meet.

If you root your daily existence in fear, anxiety, stress, worry, doubt, and terror, then you aren't living in the moment. You're living in a potential future that hasn't come to pass, convinced that you *know* what will happen and you *know* it will be *just awful.* You are no longer living; you're existing. Such thinking errors are the traps that lead people to a lifestyle of addiction and destruction in the first place.

Consider all the years you spent entering addiction. Consider all the behaviors you learned, including the criminal thinking and criminal tools you picked up along the way. Think about how you learned how to lie, cheat, steal, deceive, misdirect, play word games, and act in unscrupulous ways. You spent years perfecting what we call "Wrong Living." You mastered the workings of the person who lives his life wrong, makes wrong choices, and engages in wrong behaviors, and the outcomes are always bad.The alternative is called Right Living. Right Living embodies virtuous decisions that are rooted in pro-social behavior. Right Living takes practice. If you ask someone, "What is the right thing to do?" most people will be able to tell you. But if you ask someone to put the right way of doing things into practice, some people will still do it wrong, even after they've explained to you how to do it right! This might sound crazy, but we sometimes do these crazy things. We justify, rationalize, minimize our behaviors, blame-shift, and take a victim stance all because doing the right thing takes more effort. This is where many people get into trouble and enter Wrong Living.

Most people who abuse substances—not all, but most—will say they started abusing the drugs because of "XYZ," which means they have a *reason* why. They have rationalized why they needed to abuse substances. They might point out how wrong others are for abusing substances, but the client will justify his own behaviors. Usually when we talk with someone who abuses opiates, we hear he started taking them because of pain. When someone abuses alcohol, we usually hear something about how it helped her unwind. People who talk about abusing methamphetamines often say they just wanted some extra energy or wanted to feel good. In short, everyone has a reason why they abuse substances.

Yet, if you ask these same people, "What steps did you take that were safe, legal, and healthy to address the problems you had?" we'll hear how they went to a doctor, or how they had legal prescriptions but didn't like the side effects, or how it would have been too hard, taken too long, etc.

Therefore, they took a shortcut to getting something to alter their moods.

Of course, we can demonstrate how these ways of thinking and behaving led the client down the path of Wrong Living. The biggest thing to note is that Right Living takes an effort. It takes practice. It requires a sense of integrity and personal code of conduct that involves applied wisdom. Wisdom, for the record, is not the same thing as intelligence. Intelligence is knowing what is Right Living and what is Wrong Living. Wisdom is the ability to put that intelligence into practice. Wisdom is applied intelligence. Right Living, therefore, requires you to draw upon your smarts and your willpower simultaneously. That's difficult; it takes work.

It's easy to get off on the wrong path. We give in to our instant gratification because we want to feel good *now*! We want to stop feeling pain *now*! We demand to be treated specially and not follow the rules of society because we matter the most. It becomes about *me*, and everything else—rules, laws, principles, morals, and ethics—becomes meaningless. "Heroin is illegal? Tough. I need to stop being in pain right here, right now, and I don't care if I break laws to get my fix." Instant gratification often is in opposition to wisdom. You cannot have instant gratification if wisdom screams at you, "Do not do this; you know how badly this will end."

It's hard.

But you've made so much progress so far!

You went to treatment.

You graduated from treatment.

You've set up aftercare.

You've set up sober support networks.

You're reading (and re-reading) this book.

You have names, phone numbers, and email addresses of additional supports if needed.

Look at how many tools you have at your disposal to engage in Right Living! You have set yourself up for success, and you probably haven't even thought about that.

We'd like to leave you with a final thought process that we hope will help you on your journey. We'd like to remind you that you are an expert on your own behavior. You can dread the future and you can be scared of the future. We'll support you in this and tell you it's OK to have those feelings and thoughts. But, *you alone determine what choices you will make.* Therefore, no matter how awful you think things might turn out, you already know your strengths, your areas of need, your areas of complete confusion, and so on. When situations present to you, you know how you'll respond. No matter what choice you plan to make, you know the choice is yours. You made a choice when you entered treatment; now that you've left treatment, every choice is still yours from here on out. No one will make you choose; *you* will choose.

Imagine a sober tomorrow. Tomorrow, imagine it again while you're living it.

We hope you'll let us know how well your life is going!

BIBLIOGRAPHY

Dorsman, Jerry. *How to Quit Drinking Without AA*. Roseville, CA: Prima, 1997.

Ellis, Albert, and Emmet Velten. *When AA Doesn't Work: Rational Steps to Quitting Alcohol*. Fort Lee, NJ: Barricade, 1992.

Fletcher, Anne M. *Inside Rehab: The Surprising Truth About Addiction Treatment – And How to Get Help That Works*. New York: Viking, 2013.

————. *Sober for Good: New Solutions for Drinking Problems—Advice from Those Who Have Succeeded*. New York: Houghton Mifflin Harcourt, 2002.

Hardin, Rosemary. *SMART Recovery Handbook* (3rd Edition). Mentor, OH: Alcohol and Drug Abuse Self Help Network, 2013.

Heyman, Gene M. *Addiction: A Disorder of Choice*. Cambridge: Harvard University Press, 2010.

Marlatt, Alan, and Deborah Romaine. *The Complete Idiot's Guide to Changing Old Habits for Good*. New York: Penguin, 2008.

Peele, Stanton. *Diseasing of America: How We Allowed Recovery Zealots and the Treatment Industry to Convince Us We Are Out of Control*. San Francisco: Jossey-Bass, 1999.

Peele, Stanton, and Archie Brodsky. *The Truth About Addiction and Recovery*. New York: Touchstone, 1992.

Perkins, Cynthia. *Get Sober Stay Sober: The Truth About Alcoholism*. Yucca Valley, CA: Cynthia Perkins Publications, 2009.

Pescosolido, Bernice A., Jack K. Martin, Scott Long, Tait Medina, Jo C. Phelan, and Bruce Link. "A Disease Like Any Other? A Decade of Change in Public Relations to Schizophrenia, Depression and Alcohol Dependence," *American Journal of Psychiatry* (2010), 167(11): 1321–1330.

Soderman, Peter, and Michael Werner. *Powerless No Longer: Reprogramming Your Addictive Behavior*. Charleston: CreateSpace, 2013.

Spiegelman, Erica. *Rewired: A Bold New Approach to Addiction and Recovery*. Hobart, NY: Hatherleigh, 2015.

Szalavitz, Maia. *Unbroken Brain: A Revolutionary New Way of Understanding Addiction*. New York: St. Martin's, 2016.

Tate, Philip. *Alcohol: How to Give It Up and Be Glad You Did*. Tucson: Sharp, 1996.

Trimpey, Jack. *Rational Recovery: The New Cure for Substance Addiction*. New York: Gallery, 1996.